Ophthalmic Medications and Pharmacology

Second Edition

Brian Duvall, OD
Snoqualamie Valley Eyecare
North Bend, Washington

Robert M. Kershner, MD, MS, FACS
Eye Laser Consulting
Boston, Massachusetts

Series Editors:
Janice K. Ledford • Ken Daniels • Robert Campbell

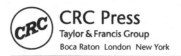

CRC Press
Taylor & Francis Group
Boca Raton London New York

CRC Press is an imprint of the
Taylor & Francis Group, an **informa** business

First published 2006 by SLACK Incorporated

Published 2024 by CRC Press
2385 NW Executive Center Drive, Suite 320, Boca Raton FL 33431

and by CRC Press
4 Park Square, Milton Park, Abingdon, Oxon, OX14 4RN

CRC Press is an imprint of Taylor & Francis Group, LLC

Library of Congress Cataloging-in-Publication Data

Duvall, Brian, 1968-
   Ophthalmic medications and pharmacology / Brian Duvall, Robert
M. Kershner. -- 2nd ed.
     p. ; cm.
   Includes bibliographical references and index.
   ISBN-13: 9781556427503 (alk. paper)
   1. Ocular pharmacology.   I. Kershner, Robert M., 1953-
II. Title.
   [DNLM: 1. Eye Diseases--drug therapy. 2. Ophthalmic Solutions
--pharmacology.   WW 166 D983o 2006]
   RE994.D88 2006
   617.7'061--dc22
                                2005020695

ISBN: 9781556427503 (pbk)
ISBN: 9781003525394 (ebk)

DOI: 10.1201/9781003525394

Dedication

This book is dedicated to our patients, who are our single greatest resource for continuing education and professional satisfaction.

A book of this magnitude takes hundreds of hours of work and preparation, time that is spent away from our families and loved ones. It is with the love and understanding of our wives, Latreash Duvall and Jeryl Kershner, that we dedicate this book.

Dedication

Contents

Contents

Acknowledgments

In an undertaking such as this, so much work is done unseen so that I may receive credit. I wish to give credit back to all those individuals, in particular, Jan Ledford, who handled, guided, and shaped this text along its journey to completion, and Dr. Robert Kershner for his effort, knowledge, and willingness to share this opportunity so many years ago.

Thanks also to all those whose knowledge, guidance, and friendship have been so instrumental in my life and career: Drs. Leland Carr, Michael Orr, George Pardos, Robert Prouty, Alan Reichow, David Souza, Debra Stone, my mentors and teachers, and the wonderful staffs that I have been privileged to know and work with. I'd also like to thank my parents, Gary and Sandy, as well as Linda and Mike, Gary and Nani, and the rest of my family and friends.

Lastly, I acknowledge and give thanks to the Lord for all the special blessings I have received — my children Ethan, Lauren, and Luke — and especially for the one lady with whom the joy I feel will never be surpassed: my wife, Latreash.

— Brian Duvall, OD

This book is the culmination of many hours of hard work—writing, dictating, transcribing, and, finally, publishing. I would like to thank my colleague, Brian S. Duvall, OD, who spent literally hundreds of hours researching and writing to keep this book as comprehensive and up-to-date as possible. My thanks to the pharmaceutical companies who strive to produce newer and better pharmacologic agents, which provide us, as the practitioners of eyecare, an ever-expanding armamentarium with which to treat a wide range of eye diseases. A special acknowledgment to my family—my wife, Jeryl, and my daughters, Shaina and Emily.

— Robert M. Kershner, MD, MS, FACS

About the Authors

Brian S. Duvall, OD, pursued his undergraduate studies at Central Washington University and his Doctor of Optometry from Pacific University College of Optometry, graduating with distinction. Dr. Duvall then completed fellowship training in the treatment and management of ocular disease at Omni Eye Specialist in Denver, Colo. Following his residency training, Dr. Duvall served in Tucson, Ariz as the Director of Optometric Consultative services at The Orange Grove Center for Corrective Eye Surgery. With the emergence of excimer laser technology, Dr. Duvall joined TLC Laser Eye Centers as an Executive and Clinical Director in both Indianapolis and Seattle, serving as a consultant, clinician, and educator. Dr. Duvall currently serves as director at Snoqualmie Valley Eyecare, a private group practice in the Cascade gateway, east of Seattle, Wash.

Aside from his clinical and administrative duties, Dr. Duvall maintains his role as an educator and consultant within the optometric community; he lectures and publishes frequently on many aspects of medical and surgical eyecare and has served as co-host with Dr. Kershner on television's "Eye on Health." Dr. Duvall has volunteered his time and resources on eyecare mission trips, has served at many levels in his local and state organizations, and is an adjunct Professor to Pacific University College of Optometry. Dr. Duvall has received the highest accolades from faculty, students, patients, and colleagues as an accomplished educator and clinician. The role he cherishes most is that of husband to his wife Latreash and father to their 3 children.

Robert M. Kershner, MD, MS, FACS, pursued his undergraduate studies in Molecular Biology at Boston University, graduated with honors, and received the Distinguished Alumni Award in 2002. He received his Masters of Science in Cell Biology and Biochemistry and Doctor of Medicine degrees with honors at the University of Vermont College of Medicine. He completed his Internship in General Surgery and his specialty training in Ophthalmology at the University of Arizona Health Sciences Center in Tucson, and was chief resident in Ophthalmology at the University of Utah Medical Center in Salt Lake City, Utah.

He is certified by the American Board of Ophthalmology, subspecialty certified in Cataract and Refractive Surgery by the American Board of Eye Surgery, a Fellow of the American Academy of Ophthalmology, a Fellow of the American Society of Cataract and Refractive Surgery, and a Fellow of the American College of Surgeons. Dr. Kershner is President and CEO of Eye Laser Consulting, Boston, Mass; Clinical Professor of Ophthalmology at the John A. Moran Eye Center, University of Utah School of Medicine in Salt Lake City, Utah; IK Ho Visiting Professor of Ophthalmology at the Chinese University of Hong Kong; Past Chief of the Section of Ophthalmology and nominated for Chief of Staff at Northwest Medical Center, Tucson, Ariz; Past Medical Director-Pima Medical Institute; Board Member, American College of Eye Surgeons; Past Chairman of the Anterior Segment Fellowship Program; and Founder and *Director Emeritus* of the Eye Laser Center in Tucson, Ariz.

Dr. Kershner has authored over 200 scientific articles, contributed to 20 textbooks, and is on the editorial board of numerous scientific journals. He has been featured on radio, in print (in *USA Today* and *Newsweek*, performing surgery with the Implantable Miniature Telescope), and on television (on *CNN* and *ABC's Evening News Tonight with Peter Jennings,* as well as hosting the popular weekly cable television series "Eye on Health").

Dr. Kershner has been active in research to develop new intraocular lens implants, is a pioneer in the development of new microsurgical techniques (for cataract, refractive, and glaucoma surgery), and has developed numerous medical devices and surgical instruments that bear his name.

In addition to teaching other ophthalmologists and industry representatives in the United States, Dr. Kershner has been an invited speaker in Austria, Brazil, France, Italy, Norway, India, Canada, Mexico, China, Switzerland, Thailand, Taiwan, Japan, South Africa, Holland, Australia, Czech Republic, and Russia. He has been honored for his teaching and surgical skills by the International Association for Training and Research in Ophthalmic Surgery in Stansstad, Switzerland; by the late Director General and Professor Svyatoslav N. Fyodorov of the Intersectoral Research and Technology Complex in Moscow, Russia; and by the Japanese Society for Cataract Research, the Japan Intraocular Lens Implant Society. He is the recipient of the Alcon Surgical Award for Achievement in Ophthalmology, the Achievement Award of the American Academy of Ophthalmology, the gold medal from the Indian Intraocular Implant and Refractive Society (the Maharshtra Ophthalmic Society, the Bombay Ophthalmologist's Association), and received the IK HO Visiting Professorship of Ophthalmology from the Chinese University of Hong Kong. In 1994, Dr. Kershner received the Republican Senatorial Medal of Freedom, the highest honor the Republican members of the United States Senate can bestow on a private citizen.

Dr. Kershner was listed in the 2002-2003 *Guide to America's Top Ophthalmologists* published by the Consumers' Research Council of America in Washington, DC. He received a National Leadership Award given by Dennis Hastert, Speaker of the House, on behalf of the United States Congress in 2002. He was inducted into the Collegium of Distinguished Alumni of the College of Arts and Sciences at Boston University in May 2002. He continues his research, writing, and lecturing, and lives with his wife (who is a physician) and daughters in Boston.

Introduction

The field of drug therapy is a rapidly changing and somewhat bewildering area to study. In developing and writing this textbook, we consulted the most up-to-date sources for information on new drug therapies. No textbook can be complete, especially when it covers an area as vast as the field of ocular pharmacology and therapeutics. Nonetheless, we have made a conscientious effort to cover the most important and commonly used medications in a format that is easy to read. We hope that this textbook will serve you well as a reference in reviewing different classes of drugs, their dosages, therapeutic uses, and potential side effects. As no textbook can ever be complete and immediately up-to-date, we encourage you to supplement this text with the latest volume of the *Physician's Desk Reference*, especially the supplements on ophthalmology and nonprescription drugs, published by Thomson Healthcare, Montvale, NJ.

We feel that our collaborative efforts representing the fields of optometry and ophthalmology bring to this book 2 important and complementary points of view in the pharmacological treatment of eye diseases. We hope that you find this a valuable resource and will consult it frequently.

Brian S. Duvall, OD
Consultative Optometry

Robert M. Kershner, MD, MS, FACS
Ophthalmic Surgeon

The Study Icons

The *Basic Bookshelf For Eyecare Professionals* is quality educational material designed for professionals in all branches of eyecare. Because so many of you want to expand your careers, we have made a special effort to include information needed for certification exams. When these study icons appear in the margin of a *Series* book, it is your cue that the material next to the icon is listed as a criteria item for a certification examination. Please use this key to identify the appropriate icon:

OptP	paraoptometric
OptA	paraoptometric assistant
OptT	paraoptometric technician
OphA	ophthalmic assistant
OphT	ophthalmic technician
OphMT	ophthalmic medical technologist[*]
Srg	ophthalmic surgical assisting subspecialty
CL	contact lens registry
Optn	opticianry
RA	retinal angiographer[†]

[*]Note: Because this icon applies to the entire book, it will not appear anywhere on the pages.

[†]Note: The criteria for certification as a retinal angiographer lists "Pharmacology" without any further breakdown of this complex topic. Therefore this icon will not appear in this text.

Chapter 1

Pharmaceutical Characteristics and Delivery

KEY POINTS

- In addition to the drug, pharmaceutical preparation has added ingredients to control pH, tonicity, viscosity, and microbial contamination.

- Pharmaceutical breakdown occurs as a result of extreme temperature, moisture, and light. Store pharmaceuticals to avoid these factors.

- Preservatives are used to control microbial contamination. They can, however, cause corneal toxicity in some patients.

- Anterior segment conditions are normally treated topically. In addition to being more effective, topical medications also avoid the increased risks and side effects of systemic administration.

Pharmaceutical agents are used daily for patient evaluation, diagnosis, and treatment. Many patients are also using other drugs to treat various medical conditions. A general understanding of pharmacology, therapeutics, drug administration, makeup, actions, interactions, and side effects is critical for those involved in patient care.

Originally, physicians prepared their own pharmaceutical agents. Today, most, if not all, pharmaceuticals are prepared commercially. This ensures uniformity and sterility of the preparations. The technicalities of drug preparation fall into the realm of the pharmacist. However, physicians and other health care providers should still understand how medications are prepared.

A number of factors maximize the effectiveness and availability of modern drug preparations while minimizing potential side effects. Such factors include pH, tonicity, stability, and sterility.

pH

The measure of the acidity and alkalinity of a substance is known as the pH. A substance with a pH of less than 7 is considered acidic while those above 7 are considered alkaline (or base). The pH of the ocular tear film is approximately 7.4. Solutions with a pH below 6.6 or above 7.8 are uncomfortable when instilled into the eye. Buffers are chemicals added to a drug formulation that help to maintain a comfortable pH between 6 and 8. Alteration of the pH can have an impact on the drug's activity, however. Certain drugs penetrate the cornea more easily if the pH is elevated. Yet, this same increase in pH can decrease the stability and solubility of the drug. Drug manufacturers must find a balance between these 2 factors to maximize the desired form and function of each pharmaceutical.

Tonicity

Tonicity is the relative measure of the osmotic pressures exerted between 2 solutions. Osmosis is a process whereby fluid is drawn across a membrane until equal concentrations are established on either side. The osmotic pressure is the pressure that develops across this membrane as a result of the fluid movement. If solutions are isotonic, equal osmotic forces exist, and there is no movement between them.

Most ophthalmic solutions are designed to be isotonic with human tears (0.9 sodium chloride equivalent). Tonicity agents, or buffers, are added to a preparation to keep it in this range. Examples of tonicity agents include glycerin, sodium, potassium chloride, and other salts.

The eye can withstand solutions ranging in tonicity from 0.6 to 1.8. Outside this range, irritation, pain, and tissue damage may result. Increasing the tonicity above the isotonic range will create a hypertonic solution. Hypertonic solutions are used if water needs to be drawn out of the eye, as in corneal edema and angle-closure glaucoma. The use of oral and topical hypertonic solutions will be discussed later.

Stability

No complex drug is indefinitely stable in solution. Pharmaceutical companies must create solutions that stay in their active form and have a shelf life long enough to withstand the time constraints of manufacturing, shipping, and storage. Drugs that are slightly acidic tend to be more stable than neutral or alkaline preparations.

Pharmaceutical degradation is aided by light, moisture, and heat. Bottle caps should always be kept tightly fastened and solutions kept at room temperature (with a few exceptions). In general, drops do not need to be refrigerated, as extreme cold or freezing may enhance breakdown. Avoid storing drugs in direct sunlight. Once opened and exposed, solutions are degraded by oxygen (oxidation). Medications should be stored in their opaque containers. Certain additives, called antioxidants, can stabilize a solution by minimizing deterioration. An example of an antioxidant is sodium bisulfate.

Sterility and Preservatives

Once opened, solutions are not only exposed to degradation but also to microbial contamination. *Pseudomonas aeruginosa* is a well-known contaminant of sodium fluorescein. *Acanthamoeba*, a protozoan, is known to invade homemade saline solutions. Unknowingly introducing one of these, or any other microbe, into the eye can have devastating results. Preservatives are added to drug preparations to control microbial growth.

Like antibiotics, preservatives are divided into 2 classes: *bacteriostatic* and *bactericidal*. Though having similar classification, antibiotics are formulated to affect specific organisms, while preservatives act against all cells. In either situation, bacteriostatic substances act to inhibit the growth of the cell, while bactericidal substances inhibit cell reproduction or kill the cell outright.

Benzalkonium chloride remains one of the most popular bacteriocidal preservatives. Although it can be rather toxic, this serves to enhance drug penetration. Thimerisol is another preservative that has been used due to its bacteriostatic properties. However, many patients developed sensitivity to it after only short periods of corneal contact. It has now been widely replaced with other agents.

In the field of artificial tears, there has been a focus on the development of less irritating preservatives. For instance, sodium perborate (Gen-aqua®) is used in Genteal®. This agent is unique in that contact with the eye changes it into oxygen and water, producing minimally-lasting negative effects. Purite (in Refresh®) and Polyquaternium-1 (in Systane®) are other new additions to the line of artificial tears preservatives. Other common preservatives include chlorbutol, phenylethyl alcohol, and sorbic acid.

Ethylenediaminetetraacetic acid is a chelating agent, or a chemical whose action increases the effectiveness of other preservatives. It, too, has been shown to cause sensitivity in some patients.

What the Patient Needs to Know

- Keep drops and ointments at room temperature unless instructed otherwise. Pockets and cars tend to have elevated temperatures, which can alter the drug's effectiveness. Extreme cold may also cause the drug to degrade.

- To preserve sterility, do not touch the dropper tip to the lashes, lids, or fingers. Do not set the cap on a countertop.

Vehicles

Vehicles are inert (nonactive) agents that either provide support for or are used to dissolve the active drug. Though they may be used as a buffer, their major function is to control viscosity (thickness) of the solution. Increasing the viscosity increases the contact time of the active drug. Some commonly used vehicles in ophthalmic solutions are povidone (PVP), polyvinyl alcohol, and carboxymethylcellulose. To increase contact time, certain ophthalmic preparations use special gel-forming vehicles. One of these, Gelrite® (in Timoptic XE®), allows the medication to remain in solution until it contacts the precorneal tear film. It then forms a more viscous gel, which is subsequently removed by the tears over time. Finally, vehicles such as white petrolatum and lanolin are used in ophthalmic ointments.

Excipients

Excipients are inactive substances that are added to give form or consistency to the preparation. Salts, sugars, fillers, binders, lubricants (as an additive), colors, and flavors fall into this group. They have limited use and application in ophthalmic medications.

Drug Administration

There are several routes of drug administration, each suitable for given conditions. Although different ocular conditions can be treated in a variety of ways, the best method is always a combination of a) the most effective route for the condition and the tissue (ie, topical, local, or systemic), b) the method that will be easiest for the patient to comply with, and c) the drug and route that has the least risk and the lowest possibility of side effects.

Topical

Ophthalmic drugs must reach the eye in high concentrations. Many systemic medications do not penetrate the anterior segment due to the blood aqueous barrier. When the desired target is the cornea, conjunctiva, ciliary body, or other anterior segment structures, topical administration is best. Topical administration involves placing the drug in contact with the surface tissues of the eye by use of solutions, suspensions, ointments, gels, and other means. The drug then passes through the cornea or conjunctiva and is carried to the intended site.

Solutions and Suspensions

Most topical pharmaceuticals are in the form of solutions or suspensions. Solutions contain the active drug dissolved in a liquid medium. In a suspension, the drug is very finely divided and suspended (not dissolved) in a liquid medium. When a suspension is allowed to sit, the solid drug will sink to the bottom of the container. Suspensions must be shaken prior to use to resuspend the particles and ensure that the proper amount of drug is delivered to the eye.

What the Patient Needs to Know

- When a suspension is prescribed, shake the bottle before using.

Solutions and suspensions are used frequently because they are easy to install and have fewer potential complications. However, solutions and suspensions have a relatively short contact time, somewhat imprecise delivery, and are easily contaminated.

Ointments

Ointments are also very popular in ophthalmic practice. In ointments, the active drug is combined with a vehicle that melts when it contacts the eye. The ointment then slowly spreads out, and the drug is released. In this way, contact time is increased. However, increased contact time may increase the likelihood of allergic reaction. There are also concerns that the use of ointments may delay corneal wound healing, though this is widely debated. Another point of interest is that ointments, on rare occasions, have become entrapped within the healing cornea. This situation resolves itself, and no treatment is necessary. Because these medications blur the vision, they are best instilled when visual difficulties are least likely to cause impairment (eg, at bedtime).

What the Patient Needs to Know

- To instill ointment, gently pull your lower lid down to create a pocket. Place a small ribbon of ointment (about one-fourth inch) into the pocket, and close your eyes for a minute, allowing the medication to melt.

- Ointment or gel will blur your vision. Do not use before driving. If your physician approves, use ointment before going to bed or at another such time when the blurring will not be a problem.

Gels

To improve patient compliance and to decrease the need for multiple drops, some drugs have been formulated as gels (such as Pilopine-HS® gel) or gel-forming sustained release preparations (such as Timoptic XE®). The active drug in these preparations is released more slowly, prolonging its effect. Like ointments, they will blur the vision.

Other Topical Routes

Soft contact lenses and collagen shields can be used to deliver topical preparations. After soaking in the appropriate solution (usually an antibiotic), the lens is inserted and acts as a drug reservoir. Thus, the drug has increased contact time and prolonged release. However, contact lenses must be used with caution, as bacteria can bind to the lens matrix and precipitate an infection.

Strips

Ophthalmic dyes, such as sodium fluorescein and rose bengal, are available in single application filter paper strips. When placed in contact with the eye or moistened with a sterile solution, the dye is released from the strip. After use, the strip is discarded. These strips have proven useful due to cleanliness, convenience, and low rate of contamination.

Sprays

There have been attempts to administer drugs, such as cycloplegics and mydriatics, via sprays. This would seem advantageous in situations where apprehension interferes with application, particularly in children. The spray can be applied to the closed eyelids, and then the patient is instructed to blink, allowing the drug to enter the eye. There seems to be less irritation to the eye with this route. However, no routinely used ophthalmic drug is available in spray form at this time, though preparations can be formulated by certain pharmacies.

Local Administration/Injections

Some conditions affecting the lids, orbit, or posterior segment require concentrations of drugs greater than what is obtainable with topical administration. In these cases, local injection is an option. Injections place larger concentrations of the active drug directly at the desired location. The drug is then carried by simple diffusion into the surrounding tissues and through adjacent blood vessels.

In a subconjunctival injection, the drug is injected just under the conjunctiva. If the drug is injected beneath Tenon's capsule, it is called a sub-Tenon's injection. These methods are commonly used when administering antibiotics. Retrobulbar injections may also be used, in which case the injection is given behind the eye. Retrobulbar injections are commonly used to anesthetize the nerves and muscles of the eyes prior to surgery.

Injecting drugs directly into the anterior chamber is called intracameral. This method is used in cases of endophthalmitis, a potentially blinding infection within the eye. It is not commonly used otherwise, as the drugs are often toxic to the corneal endothelium.

With all injections, there is increased risk compared with topical routes. Generally, the deeper the injection is placed, the greater the possibility of complications, such as perforation of the globe and hemorrhage. Blindness and even death can result.

Systemic Administration

Some drugs can only be administered systemically. Because of the extensive blood supply to the lids, orbit, and posterior segment, drugs given via local injection can dissipate rapidly. In these cases, venous or oral administration can be highly effective and is often the route of choice. Drugs given in these ways have the potential to affect the body's entire system. Side effects and drug interactions increase markedly when drugs are administered systemically.

Intravenous Injection

Intravenous injections (IVs) release the drug directly into the blood stream. IVs are routinely used during intraocular surgery. In cases of endophthalmitis, antibiotics are given through this route. During an angle-closure glaucoma attack, IV drugs are used to help lower the intraocular pressure (IOP). IVs are also used in administering sodium fluorescein for the photographic diagnosis of retinal disorders.

Oral Administration

Orally administered medications are absorbed through the stomach and/or the intestines. They then make their way via the blood stream to where they are needed. Oral medications are used in instances where topical medications are not effective or when it is suspected or known that an eye condition has a systemic cause. An example of the latter is where oral antibiotics are used to treat serious eyelid infections or where oral steroids are given for the treatment of Graves' disease. Oral medications are also used in some cases of severe glaucoma.

Chapter 2

Clinical Administration

History

The benefits of pharmacologic agents to the physician and patient are undeniable. However, inappropriate or accidental use or improper combinations of drugs can be detrimental or harmful. For this reason, a thorough case history must be undertaken before any drug is applied to or prescribed for the patient. This history must include a comprehensive list of all medications the patient is currently using—topical and systemic, prescribed and over-the-counter—along with their frequency and duration. A knowledge of these will help avoid problems as well as formulate the best plan of evaluation and treatment regimen. A comprehensive look at the patient's overall systemic and ocular health history should also be included because any existing condition may alter the therapeutic or diagnostic plan of attack.

Patient Evaluation

Once a comprehensive history and other pertinent information are gathered, the actual exam begins. Realize, however, that any drug introduced into the eye can affect subsequent tests. The order of tests in an ophthalmic examination can greatly impact the results. The following format (adapted from Bartlett and Jaanus) illustrates the necessity for knowledge and foresight in formulating an exam sequence.

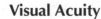

Visual Acuity

For medicolegal reasons alone, visual acuity must be the first test performed before all others. Any agent administered to the eye has the potential to adversely affect visual acuity. The acuity of each eye must, therefore, be taken prior to any other test.

Pupil Evaluation

A good pupillary evaluation is the cornerstone for assessing optic nerve function. This must be done before any mydriatic, cycloplegic, mitotic, or other pharmacologic agent is administered. Otherwise, the assessment of true pupillary function will be impeded.

Manifest Refraction

Just as any agent may potentially alter the visual acuity, the same is true for the manifest refraction. If acuity is altered, subjective response may also be affected. Cycloplegic and mydriatic drugs, in particular, affect the accommodative system. Any near point testing must then be done before dilation. If cycloplegic refraction is warranted, it should be done only after accommodative and convergence testing.

Binocular Testing

Accommodation and convergence functions are linked together. As a result, all binocular testing should be performed before cycloplegia. This includes initial cover testing and other phoria/tropia measurements. If accommodation is taken out of the picture, results can be changed drastically.

Anterior Segment Evaluation

Many drugs, particularly the anesthetics, cause degradation of the corneal epithelium. Also, the introduction of dyes can interfere with the initial appearance of the ocular surface tissues. Specifically, sodium fluorescein can permeate into the anterior chamber, hindering evaluation. Further, certain mydriatics can induce the appearance of cells in the aqueous, giving the false impression of inflammation. Finally, the instillation of drops (especially those that sting, such as anesthetics and mydriatics) can excite reflex tearing. Tear evaluation should be done before any eye drops are administered.

Tonometry

Angle-closure glaucoma is possible when patients with narrow anterior chamber angles are dilated. Assessment of the angle and a baseline IOP are required before dilation.

Drug Nomenclature

To avoid mishap, all pharmaceuticals must be properly identified. Misidentification could result in inadvertent administration of the wrong drug. Before administering any drug, make a conscious effort to read the label of every product. Many containers and product labels look similar. Do not be fooled. At first glance, people tend to see what they *expect* to see. Be aware!

To properly identify pharmaceutical agents, the physician and technician must be familiar with drug nomenclature, not only the generic but the proprietary names as well. With the thousands of prescription and nonprescription drugs available, this can be a Herculean task. For example, the commonly used antibiotic solution sodium sulfacetamide 10% is also known by the proprietary names of AK-SULF® (Akorn Pharmaceuticals), Bleph-10 Liquifilm® (Allergan), Ocusulf-10® (Optoaptics), Ophthacet® (VorTech), Sodium Sulamyd® (Schering), Sulf-10® (Iolab), and Sulten-10® (Bausch & Lomb).

You will readily become familiar with those agents used frequently in your practice, and you will gradually be able to add to your knowledge base. However, as important as knowing the drug names is knowing where to find more information about them. There are many references available that provide names, identification, and other vital information (Table 2-1).

For ease in drug identification, there has been an attempt to color code the caps of the various drugs based on the class to which they belong. Mydriatics and cycloplegics (used for dilation) have red caps. Beta-blockers (used to treat glaucoma) have yellow or blue caps. Miotics, such as pilocarpine, have green caps. Gray has been adopted as the color for nonsteroidal anti-inflammatory drugs (NSAIDs), and anti-infectives are to be identified with brown. However, this color scheme has not been universally adopted and implemented. Remember, **there is no substitute for reading the label**.

Always check the expiration date and coloration of the solution if it can be viewed. Any evidence of drug degradation or expiration signals that a preparation should be discarded.

Compliance

Patient compliance is the key to proper therapy. The physician may identify and offer a treatment plan for a given problem, but unless the patient follows the prescribed regimen, the

---

Table 2-1
Drug Information Sources

Printed References
>   *Drug Facts and Comparisons*
>   *Physicians' Desk Reference*
>   *FDC Reports*
>   *The Merck Index*
>   *Martindale: The Complete Drug Reference*
>   *Drug Induced Ocular Side Effects*
>   *Drug Interactions*
>   Other ophthalmic literature (texts, journals, etc)

Internet References
>   www.rxlist.com
>   www.medicineonline.com
>   http://www.accessdata.fda.gov/scripts/cder/drugsatfda/index.cfm?fuseaction=
>   Search.Search_Drug_Name
>   http://www.medsafe.govt.nz/Profs/Datasheet/datasheet.htm
>   http://www.drugs.com/
>   http://www.rxmed.com/b.main/b2.pharmaceutical/b2.prescribe.html
>   http://www.bnf.org
>   http://emc.medicines.org.uk/
>   http://www.fda.gov/cder/consumerinfo/default.htm
>   http://www.medscape.com/druginfo
>   http://www.pslgroup.com/newdrugs.htm
>   http://www.centerwatch.com/patient/drugs/druglist.html
>   http://www.rphworld.com

(Adapted from Clinical Optometric Pharmacology and Therapeutics. See Bibliography for publishers, etc)

situation may not improve. This is especially true in ophthalmic practice. It is usually up to the patient to instill medication himself. Compliance may be difficult due to apprehension, lack of dexterity, or confusion over instructions (not to mention forgetfulness, expense, or a number of other factors). The number of patients who comply exactly with a given set of instructions is estimated between 25% and 50% and may be lower. Therefore, every effort must be made to reduce the reasons for noncompliance.

There are many ways a patient may not comply. Medications may not be put in often enough, or they may be used too often in hopes of getting a greater effect. Medication may not be stored properly or may not be shaken when required. In addition, when more than one medication is thrown into the mix or multiple conditions are being treated concurrently, problems with compliance become more likely.

Education is the key. It starts with providing the patient with a basic understanding of his or her condition and its likely course. A patient with primary open-angle glaucoma, for example, must be told that this is a chronic condition that is controlled over a lifetime (not cured) and, therefore, drops must be used regularly every day. Patients must also be informed what the medications are specifically to be used for so that they are not used in a haphazard or harmful way. Normal side effects, such as stinging or bitter taste, must be explained so that when they occur, the patient is not alarmed.

Multiple drops at one time is not advisable. The conjunctival sac can hold no more than a single drop. Multiple drops will only increase unwanted side effects. The extra drops spill down the cheek, wasting drops and burdening the patient with the expense of additional prescriptions.

For medications to be effective, they must be given time to absorb. A minimum of 5 minutes (min) is required between drops if multiple drops are used. Ointments or gel preparations should always be administered last so as not to interfere with the absorption of other drugs. If this rule is not followed, the therapeutic effects may be lessened.

All patients should be given verbal and written instructions on the proper administration of eye drops and ointments. Cases have been reported where patients actually drank their eye drops. Proper education provided by the eyecare staff will greatly improve compliance, directly impacting successful treatment and patient satisfaction.

What the Patient Needs to Know

OptA
OptT
OphA

- Always check the label and expiration date of the medication before using.
- Applying more than 1 drop in the eye during a single application gives no additional benefit, and the waste can be costly.
- Allow a minimum of 5 min between drops if using more than one type of medication.
- Always use ointments or gels last.
- To instill eye drops:
  1. Tilt head back and look at ceiling.
  2. Gently pull eyelid down and away from eyeball.
  3. Instill 1 drop into exposed sac.
  4. Gently close eyes for 1 min.
- To instill eye ointment:
  1. Gently grasp lower lid and pull away from eyeball.
  2. Apply a small amount of ointment (¼" ribbon) into exposed sac.
  3. Gently close eyes.
              - OR -
  1. Apply small amount of ointment to clean fingertip.
  2. Gently pull down lower lid with opposite hand.
  3. Apply ointment directly onto exposed sac.
  4. Gently close eyes.

The Prescription

In any fundamental understanding of pharmacology, one needs the ability to decipher a written prescription. In addition to the fact that you may be required to write or interpret an "Rx," chart notes are often recorded in the same format.

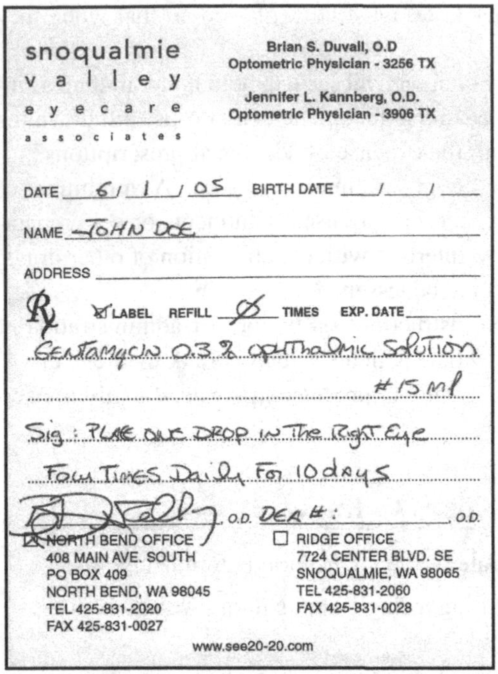

snoqualmie valley eyecare associates

Brian S. Duvall, O.D
Optometric Physician - 3256 TX

Jennifer L. Kannberg, O.D.
Optometric Physician - 3906 TX

DATE 6/1/05 BIRTH DATE __/__/__

NAME JOHN DOE

ADDRESS

℞ ☒ LABEL REFILL Ø TIMES EXP. DATE

Gentamycin 0.3% opthalmic solution
#15 ml

Sig: Place one drop in the Right Eye
Four Times Daily For 10 days

O.D. DEA #: O.D.

☒ NORTH BEND OFFICE
408 MAIN AVE. SOUTH
PO BOX 409
NORTH BEND, WA 98045
TEL 425-831-2020
FAX 425-831-0027

☐ RIDGE OFFICE
7724 CENTER BLVD. SE
SNOQUALMIE, WA 98065
TEL 425-831-2060
FAX 425-831-0028

www.see20-20.com

Figure 2-1. Typical ophthalmic prescription with written instructions.

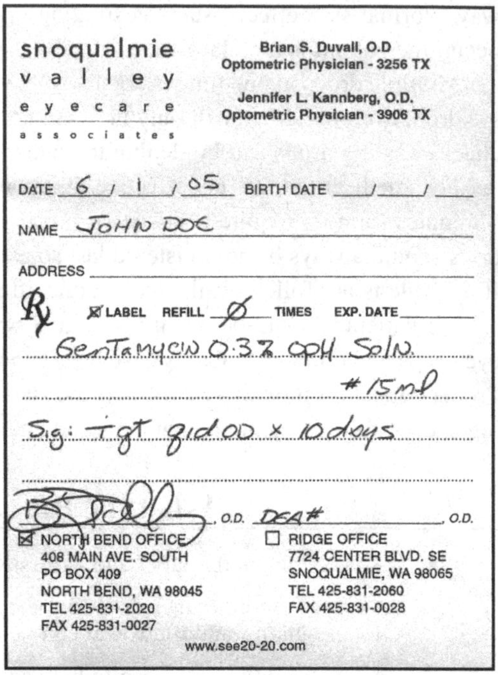

snoqualmie valley eyecare associates

Brian S. Duvall, O.D
Optometric Physician - 3256 TX

Jennifer L. Kannberg, O.D.
Optometric Physician - 3906 TX

DATE 6/1/05 BIRTH DATE __/__/__

NAME JOHN DOE

ADDRESS

℞ ☒ LABEL REFILL Ø TIMES EXP. DATE

Gentamycin 0.3% oph Soln
#15 ml

Sig: i gt qid OD x 10 days

O.D. DEA# O.D.

☒ NORTH BEND OFFICE
408 MAIN AVE. SOUTH
PO BOX 409
NORTH BEND, WA 98045
TEL 425-831-2020
FAX 425-831-0027

☐ RIDGE OFFICE
7724 CENTER BLVD. SE
SNOQUALMIE, WA 98065
TEL 425-831-2060
FAX 425-831-0028

www.see20-20.com

Figure 2-2. Same prescription as in Figure 2-1, written using classic abbreviations.

The written prescription has 4 major parts. First, there is specific physician and patient information (name, address, etc). The next section is called the inscription. This contains the name of the prescribed agent, either by generic or trade name. It also gives the concentration of the drug, if necessary. The inscription is followed by the subscription. The subscription contains the amount of drug to be dispensed by the pharmacist. This can be the exact number of tablets, the volume of solution, or the size of a tube of ointment. To avoid unwanted use following resolution of the condition, it is customary to prescribe the least amount needed. A refill can always be ordered if necessary. The last major component of the written prescription is the instructions. In its most basic form, the instructions will contain the route of administration, the number of drops or tablets to be used, and the frequency to be administered. The instructions may also contain further details, including the purpose, maximum to be used, the number of refills permitted, as well as other drugs and foods to be avoided. When it comes to writing a prescription, the more thorough, the better (Figures 2-1 and 2-2).

The specifics of a prescription are critical. They are of no use if they cannot be read. The prescription must be legible. Jokes about sloppy physician handwriting are no laughing matter when it comes to prescription writing. Illegible prescriptions can lead to misinterpretation and error on the part of the pharmacist who reads them.

The current trend is to write everything out in plain English. However, traditional abbreviations are still commonly used and will continue to be used due to habit and physician preference. Moreover, chart notes are often written using the same abbreviations. All physicians and technical help should become versed in these abbreviations. A list of the more common abbreviations can be found in Table 2-2. Whenever in doubt about a given prescription, instructions, or abbreviations, the physician responsible should be consulted to avoid misinterpretation.

Table 2-2
Common Abbreviations Used in Prescription Writing

ac	before meals
bid	twice a day
c, cum	with
Coll., Collyr	eyewash
caps	capsule
d.	day
disp.	dispense
gt(t)	drop(s)
h	hour
hs	at bedtime
OD	right eye
Oh	every hour
OS	left eye
OU	both eyes
p.c.	after meals
po	by mouth
prn	as needed
no., #	number
q	every
qh	every hour
qid	4 times a day
q2h	every 2 hours
qs	as much as needed
Rx	prescribe
s, sine	without
sig	instructions
sol	solution
susp	suspension
tab	tablet
tid	3 times a day
ung	ointment
ut dict	as directed
i	one
ii	two
iii	three

Bibliography

Bartlett JD, Jaanus SD. *Clinical Ocular Pharmacology*. 4th ed. Boston, Mass: Butterworth-Heinmann Publishing; 2001.

Catania LJ. *Primary Care of the Anterior Segment*. 2nd ed. East Norwalk, Conn: Appleton & Lange; 1996.

Drug Facts and Comparisons. Philadelphia, Pa: JB Lippincott; monthly and annual volumes.

Drug Interactions: Clinical Significance of Drug-Drug Interactions. 6th ed. Philadelphia, Pa: Lea & Febiger; 1989.

FDC Reports, Prescription and OTC Pharmaceuticals. Chevy Chase, Md: FDC Reports; published bi-weekly.

Fingeret M, Cassera L, Woodcome HT. *Atlas of Primary Eyecare Procedures*. New York, NY: McGraw-Hill Medical; 1997.

Fraunfelder FT, Grove JA, ed. *Drug Induced Ocular Side Effects*. 4th ed. Philadelphia, Pa: Lea & Febiger; 1996.

Merck Index. 13th ed. Hoboken, NJ: John Wiley & Sons; 2001.

Onefrey BE, ed. *Clinical Optometric Pharmacology and Therapeutics*. Philadelphia, Pa: JB Lippincott, Williams. & Wilkins; 1991.

Physicians' Desk Reference. (59th edition, 33rd edition for ophthalmology, 26th edition for nonprescription drugs) Montvale, NJ: Thomson PDR; published annually.

Reynolds J. *Martindales, The Extra Pharmacopoeia*. 29th ed. London, England: Pharmaceutical Riess; 1989.

Sweetman SC, ed. *Martindale: The Complete Drug Reference*. 34th ed. London, England: Pharmaceutical Press; 2004.

Chapter 3

The Autonomic Nervous System

KEY POINTS

- The autonomic nervous system consists of 2 branches: the sympathetic and parasympathetic. The actions of these 2 systems generally oppose one another.

- The sympathetic system is responsible for the excited state of the body. Pupillary dilation occurs as a result of sympathetic stimulation.

- The parasympathetic system is responsible for the body's resting state. Pupillary constriction and accommodation are a result of parasympathetic activity.

- Neurotransmitters are chemical messengers of the nervous system. Certain pharmaceuticals work by stimulating, mimicking, or inhibiting these messengers. This helps manipulate the autonomic functions.

System Divisions and Neurotransmitters

Think of your body as a large company or organization with many divisions. In any such organization, a regulating agency is needed to maintain priority and balance, or things will run amuck. In your body, the regulating agency is known as the autonomic nervous system. It oversees the systems of the body through 2 divisions. These are known as the sympathetic and parasympathetic divisions. The 2 divisions work opposite each other to maintain balance. One division causes an organ to become excited; the other division causes it to slow down.

The sympathetic nervous system is known as the "fight or flight" system because its effects are most pronounced when we are excited or find ourselves in a threatening situation. The results of increased sympathetic activity are a rapidly pounding heart; deep, rapid breathing; and dilated pupils. The blood vessels of the skin and digestive system are constricted so that blood can be made more available for the heart and skeletal muscles. All functions that are not essential to immediate survival are decreased. In the words of anatomist Elaine Mareib, RN, PhD, "When you are running from a mugger, it is far more important that your muscles be provided with everything they need to get you out of harm's way than that you finish digesting lunch."

Conversely, the parasympathetic division is concerned with the body's functions in its resting state. Its main goal is to conserve energy and promote digestion. When the parasympathetic division dominates, there is an increase in digestion, the skin is flush, pupils are constricted, and the lens of the eye accommodates for near. (Though both extremes have been illustrated here, in actuality the 2 systems work together in unison to reach a harmony and equilibrium for the stresses and activities encountered by the body at a given time).

The workings of the human nervous system are extremely complex. It involves many intertwined functions and biochemical reactions that are beyond the scope of this text. We will, however, examine it briefly for a basic understanding. First, the brain sends a command to a muscle. A signal is sent out. This signal passes through the complex network that makes up the nervous system before arriving at a specific neuron (nerve cell) at the targeted muscle. This signal is responsible for the release of a special biochemical, known as a neurotransmitter, from the end of the neuron. This neurotransmitter crosses a gap (synapse), then attaches to specific receptors (Figure 3-1). (Think of the neurotransmitter as a key that fits into a specific lock—the receptor.) These receptors are primarily located in the cardiac muscles, the smooth (involuntary) muscles of the internal organs and blood vessels, and certain glands. Once this attachment occurs, the original command is then carried out. Before a new command can be carried out by the same muscle, the neurotransmitter must be removed from the receptors to prepare for the next signal.

In practice, we use drugs to simulate the effects of both the sympathetic and parasympathetic divisions to get a specific desired effect. This can be done by stimulating, copying, or enhancing the neurotransmitter. In addition, certain actions can be stopped by inhibiting the release of the neurotransmitter, blocking its attachment to the receptors, or delaying the cleanup process (prolonging the effect of the binding).

The major neurotransmitters of the sympathetic division are epinephrine and norepinephrine. Drugs that mimic the effects of the sympathetic system are called sympathomimetic agents, also known as adrenergic agents. Phenylephrine, a drug that dilates the pupil, is one example of a sympathomimetic agent.

Drugs can also block the activities of the sympathetic system. They are called sympatho*lytic* agents. (The term *lysis* means to break down, so the suffix *-lytic* refers to the breakdown of a compound.) Because the sympathetic and parasympathetic divisions oppose one another, a drug that

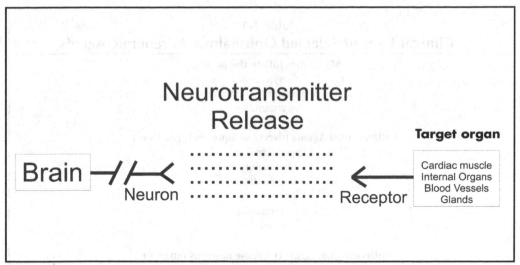

Figure 3-1. Simplified nervous system reaction.

blocks the sympathetic system will usually act like a drug that stimulates the parasympathetic system. An example of a sympatholytic agent are the beta-blockers, drugs used to control glaucoma.

The parasympathetic system uses acetylcholine as its main neurotransmitter. Drugs that mimic the effects of acetylcholine are called parasympathomimetic, or cholinergic, agents. There are also drugs that block the effects of the parasympathetic division. These are called parasympatholytic agents. Pilocarpine, another medication used in the control of glaucoma, is an example of a parasympathomimetic agent. Cyclopentolate, a cycloplegic agent, is an example of a parasympatholytic, or cholinergic-blocking, drug.

As was mentioned, the receptors also play a critical role in nerve impulse transmission. There are several types of receptors that, when bound by a neurotransmitter, can cause an increase or decrease in function. No generalization can explain the excitation or relaxation effect of a given neurotransmitter. This is determined solely by the type of receptor to which it attaches. For example, norepinephrine does not always cause contraction of blood vessels. This is determined by the type of receptor to which it binds. Certain receptor types are found more commonly in certain areas of the body. Pharmacologically, we know we can get desired effects if we can learn to target specific receptor sites.

The cholinergic receptors are divided into 2 types: *muscarinic* and *nicotinic*. Adrenergic receptors are divided into 4 types: alpha$_1$, alpha$_2$, beta$_1$, and beta$_2$. (These will be dealt with more specifically when it becomes necessary to describe certain medications later in this text.)

Cholinesterase is the chemical responsible for "cleaning up" the neurotransmitter from its attachment to the receptors. Drugs that prevent this cleanup are called anticholinesterase agents and have a sympathetic or parasympatholytic effect.

Autonomic drugs are important in ophthalmic practice due to the multitude of actions they have. Tables 3-1 and 3-2 summarize the clinical uses of the adrenergic and cholinergic drugs. Through obtaining a basic understanding of the function of the autonomic nervous system and its effects at certain sites within the body and eye, we can better understand the development, use, and side effects of the pharmaceuticals described throughout the remainder of this text. Specific

Table 3-1
Clinical Uses of Selected Ophthalmic Adrenergic Agents

Mydriatics (dilate the pupil):
phenylephrine
hydroxyamphetamine
cocaine

Antiglaucoma Agents (decrease aqueous formation):
apraclonidine
betaxolol
brimonidine
levobunolol
metipranolol
timolol

Antiglaucoma Agents (increase aqueous outflow):
epinephrine
dipivefrin

Vasoconstrictors (whiten the eye):
phenylephrine
naphazoline
oxymetazoline
tetrahydrozoline

Dilation Reversal:
dapiprazole HCl

drugs will be discussed in chapters pertaining to their appropriate clinical use. However, 2 specific autonomic drugs (which do not fit into other chapter categories) will be discussed further here: edrophonium and botulinum-A toxin.

Edrophonium

Edrophonium (Tensilon®) is occasionally used in ophthalmic practice in the diagnosis of myasthenia gravis, a neuromuscular disease causing progressive weakness and fatigue. In the eye, the symptoms can include drooping of the eyelid (ptosis). Commonly known as the Tensilon® test, a small amount of edrophonium is given intravenously. If a lid droop is due to myasthenia gravis, the drug causes a brief improvement of muscular strength, and the lid elevates. If the ptosis is not due to myasthenia, it will be unaffected by the Tensilon®.

Edrophonium is an anticholinesterase drug. Its brief duration of activity makes it ideal for diagnostic testing. Side effects are uncommon, but slowing of the heart rate and decreased blood pressure are possible. Edrophonium chloride is available in 10 ml ampules and vials ready for injection.

Table 3-2
Clinical Uses of Selected Ophthalmic Cholinergic Agents

Miotics (constrict the pupil):
pilocarpine
carbachol
physostigmine
echothiophate

Cycloplegics (paralyze accommodation):
atropine
scopolamine
homatropine
cyclopentolate
tropicamide

Diagnosis of Myasthenia Gravis:
edrophonium

Paralysis of Extraocular and Lid Muscles:
botulinum A toxin

Mydriatic Reversal:
dapiprazole

Botulinum Toxin

Botulinum toxin (Botox®) has gained widespread use primarily for cosmetic and oculoplastic procedures as well as limited use in the treatment of strabismus. Derived from a bacterial toxin, its action arises from blocking the release of acetylcholine. When injected directly into the targeted muscle, it causes a paralysis or relaxation of that muscle. Thus, it is used to relax an overactive extraocular muscle (to straighten the eye) or to calm spasms of the eyelid. The drug's maximal effect is noticed in 1 to 2 weeks but persists over a 2 to 6 month period. No systemic side effects or long-term ocular alignment problems have been reported. However, transient diplopia, blepharoptosis, and subconjunctival hemorrhages can result from botulinum toxin injection. The drug is supplied as a powder that must be reconstituted in solution for injection. It must be stored in a freezer below 23°F and is usable for 4 hours following reconstitution.

Bibliography

Bartlett JD, Jaanus SD. *Clinical Ocular Pharmacology.* 4th ed. Boston, Mass: Butterworth-Heinemann; 2001.

Caloroso EE, Rouse MW. *Clinical Management of Strabismus.* Stoneham, Mass: Butterworth-Heinemann; 1993.

Kauffman PL, Alm A. *Adler's Physiology of the Eye.* 10th ed. St. Louis, Mo: Mosby; 2003.

Marieb EN. *Human Anatomy and Physiology.* Redwood City, Ca: Benjamin/Cumming Publishing; 1989.

Moses RA, Hart WM Jr. *Adlers Physiology of Eye.* St. Louis, Mo: CV Mosby; 1987.

Onefrey BE, ed. *Clinical Optometric Pharm and Therapeutics*. Philadelphia, Pa: JB Lippincott, Williams, & Wilkins; 1991.

Ophthalmic Drug Facts. St. Louis, Mo: JB Lippincott; 1990.

Physicians Desk Reference. 59th ed. (33rd edition for ophthalmology, 26th edition for nonprescription drugs) Montvale, NJ: Thomson PDR; published annually.

von Noorden GK, Campos EC. *Binocular Vision and Ocular Motility, Theory and Management of Strabismus*. 6th ed. St. Louis, Mo: CV Mosby; 2002.

Chapter 4

Diagnostic Pharmaceuticals

- Mydriatics dilate the pupil. Cycloplegics dilate the pupil and suspend accommodation.

- Tropicamide is the drug of choice for routine dilation. It is often combined with phenylephrine or hydroxyamphetamine for added effect.

- Cyclopentolate is the drug of choice for routine cycloplegia.

- Topical ophthalmic dyes should be instilled only after evaluation of the cornea and anterior chamber, as they can alter the clinical picture.

Mydriasis vs. Cycloplegia

Mydriasis is dilation of the pupil. Drugs that act only to dilate the pupil are known as mydriatics. Mydriatics are used for diagnostic evaluation and visualization of the entire posterior segment, a view that is impossible under nondilated conditions. Mydriatics are also used to allow full visualization of the lens and other ocular structures during ophthalmic surgery.

The use of cycloplegic agents accomplishes several things. First, they dilate the pupil for ocular health assessment. Secondly, and primarily, cycloplegic agents cause paralysis of the ciliary muscle. This paralysis is called cycloplegia, which gives these agents their name.

Cycloplegia is advantageous in a number of instances. First, it lessens or eliminates the accommodative function. This is helpful in evaluating patients with latent hyperopia, accommodative esotropia, or in assessing the refractive error before refractive surgery. Cycloplegia is also desired in cases of trauma or inflammation where spasms of the ciliary muscle cause considerable eye ache and photophobia. The dilating ability of cycloplegics, in these cases, is also helpful in preventing formation of posterior synechiae (an adhesion between the iris and anterior lens capsule).

When dilated or cyclopleged, the patient will notice increased glare and photosensitivity. Depth perception may also be impaired. Patients who are cyclopleged will lose their ability to focus up close. The duration of this disability depends on the specific drug used. Sometimes, cycloplegics and mydriatics are used in combination to achieve maximum dilation greater than with either agent used alone. Often phenylephrine 2.5% and tropicamide 1% are teamed up for this purpose. Remember that all cycloplegic and mydriatic drops have red caps for easy identification.

Mydriatics

Mydriatic drugs exert their effect on the iris musculature to dilate the eye. Mydriatics have little to no effect on the accommodative function, instead stimulating the dilating muscle of the iris and sparing the ciliary musculature. All patients who are to undergo dilation must first have the anterior chamber angle depth evaluated to ascertain the risk of angle closure. As with all topical ocular medication, punctal occlusion should be used to avoid systemic effects, especially with children, the elderly, and in the presence of certain medical conditions. Caution must be taken when performing other activities while eyes remain dilated.

What the Patient Needs to Know

- All mydiatics/cycloplegics sting upon instillation.

- All mydiatics/cycloplegics have a red cap.

- Blurred vision will persist beyond exam. Caution must be taken when driving or performing other activities while eyes remain dilated.

- Sunglasses should always be worn outside when eyes are dilated to protect the retina.

- Patients at risk should be made aware of symptoms of angle closure: pain, headache, nausea, halos around lights, and decreased vision.

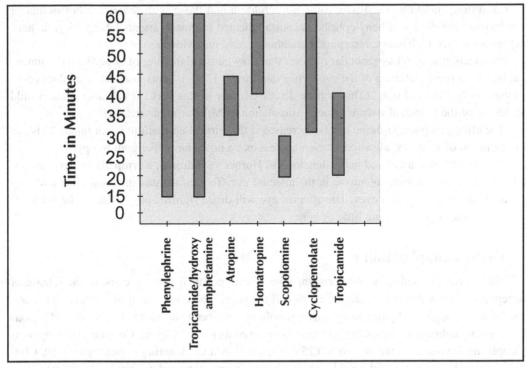

Figure 4-1. Time to maximum mydriasis.

Phenylephrine

Phenylephrine (Neo-synephrine®, Mydfrin®) is a sympathomimetic that acts to stimulate iris dilation. Normally, maximum dilation occurs about 45 to 60 min after instillation (Figure 4-1). The pupil should return to predrug size in 4 to 6 hours. The physician and technician must be aware, however, that these times can vary significantly. Diabetic patients historically tend to dilate more slowly and less widely than other patients. Also, the drug tends to bind to pigment. This means that in dark-eyed individuals, the drug does not reach its desired site in the same quantity and stays around much longer. People with dark eyes, therefore, dilate more slowly and stay dilated longer. The same is true in patients with a large anterior chamber reaction, such as iritis.

Patients will remain dilated for several hours following their examination. This may cause blurred vision. Precautions must be taken when driving or performing other activities. Patients may be told beforehand to bring a driver if dilation is to be performed. Also, because the pupils remain dilated, sunglasses should be worn when going outside both to protect the retina and for patient comfort. Mydriatic glasses should be supplied to the patients if they do not have sunglasses of their own.

Commercially, phenylephrine is available in 2.5% and 10% solutions. Recent studies have questioned the increased efficacy of the 10% versus the 2.5% solution. It appears that the incidence of risks and side effects increase greatly when the 10% solution is used.

Normally, transient stinging and blurred vision are the only major side effects inherent with the topical use of phenylephrine. However, in instances where the recommended dosage has been exceeded or when administered to a patient with severe cardiovascular disease, serious vascular reactions and elevation in blood pressure can result. Thus, phenylephrine, especially the

10% solution, should be used with caution in children and those with severe cardiovascular or cerebrovascular disease. Phenylephrine is contraindicated in those patients taking tricyclic antidepressants, MAO inhibitors, reserpine, guanethidine, and methyldopa.

Phenylephrine also has secondary effects that may cause blanching of superficial conjunctival blood vessels (whitening of the eye). Phenylephrine 0.125% is, thus, used as an ocular decongestant to "get the red out." (This will be discussed later in this text.) It can also cause a mild widening of the palpebral fissure through stimulation of Mueller's muscle.

The effects of phenylephrine can be increased if the corneal epithelium is not intact. This can be the result of a corneal abrasion or even normal exam procedures like gonioscopy.

Phenylephrine can be used in the diagnosis of Horner's syndrome, a sympathetic nervous system disorder that presents as miosis in the affected eye. To confirm this diagnosis, 1% phenylephrine is instilled into both eyes. The affected eye will dilate significantly, whereas the unaffected or "normal" eye will dilate little or none.

Hydroxyamphetamine

Hydroxyamphetamine is another sympathomimetic agent. It acts by causing the release of norepinephrine, which in turn causes dilation of the pupil. There is little, if any, effect on accommodation. Though 1% hydroxyamphetamine solution has been shown to have similar effects as 2.5% phenylephrine, hydroxyamphetamine is not used as a single agent. Commercially, hydroxyamphetamine has been teamed with 0.25% tropicamide, a weak acting cycloplegic agent. Clinically, it has been very useful for dilation due to its effectiveness and minimal side effects. However, the maximal dilation may not be adequate for those with diabetes or for extreme peripheral retinal evaluation. In the last decade, this product has been on and off the market several times and, as of this writing, is not available. If it should return, it will continue to be a popular diagnostic agent.

Mydriatic Reversal Drops

Dapiprazole (Rev-Eyes®) is useful in reversing the dilation induced by mydriatics, particularly Paremyd, and to a lesser extent tropicamide. Dapiprazole is a sympathomimetic blocking agent that acts by blocking the receptors of the iris dilator muscle.

Dapiprazole HCl is a sterile white powder that is soluble in water. Rev-Eyes® is commercially available in a kit consisting of 2 vials. One vial contains 25 mg of powdered dapiprazole HCl. The other contains 5 ml of dilutant. The kit also contains a dropper for instillation. The drug must be reconstituted in the supplied dilutant. Once mixed, it can be stored at room temperature for 21 days. (Clinically, it is easier to replace the solution only once a month. It appears to remain effective, though this has not been substantiated in clinical studies.)

The manufacturer recommends instilling 2 drops initially, followed by 2 more drops 5 min later. (Some physicians have cut this back to 2 applications of a single drop.) Dapiprazole has excellent activity against the mydriatics, with almost a 90% reduction in the dilation of phenylephrine after 1 hour. The results are much less dramatic against tropicamide, with only about 40% reduction after 2 hours.

The 2 major adverse reactions associated with topical administration of dapiprazole are burning and conjunctival injection. More than half of patients report significant burning after

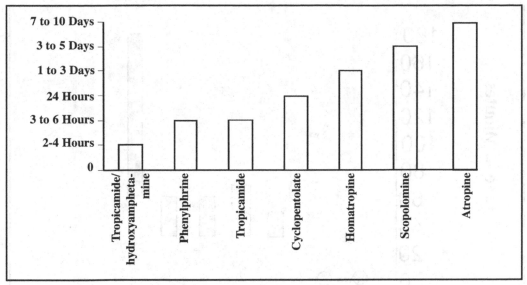

Figure 4-2. Time to mydriasis recovery.

instillation. Approximately 80% of patients have red eyes secondary to conjunctival injection after use. This redness may persist from 20 min to 1 hour.

Other cholinergic drugs, pilocarpine in particular, have been used to reverse dilation. However, this is not usually recommended due to increased risks and adverse reaction—most significantly, the risk of prompting an angle closure as a result of iris sphincter stimulation.

What the Patient Needs to Know

- Dapiprazole drops sting.
- Eyes will remain red for up to 1 hour after use.

Cycloplegic Agents

OphT

OptT

Cycloplegic agents are parasympatholytic drugs that act to block the iris sphincter and ciliary muscle. They cause dilation of the pupil and paralysis of accommodative function or cycloplegia. Cycloplegic agents are chiefly used in the refraction of children and those thought to have latent hyperopia. They are also used in dilation for fundus evaluation and in the treatment of uveal tract inflammation.

The major cycloplegic agents used today in ophthalmic practice, in order of decreasing strength, are atropine, scopolamine, homatropine, cyclopentolate, and tropicamide. Figures 4-1 through 4-4 list the times to peak mydriasis and cycloplegia as well as recovery times for these agents.

The major ocular side effects associated with instillation of cycloplegics are blurred vision and stinging. As with the mydriatics, the blurred vision is a result of the increased pupil size. In addition, though, paralysis of the accommodative system severely limits the vision at near. Understandably, this is increased when the stronger cycloplegics are used.

The use of stronger cycloplegics, particularly atropine, scopolamine, and homatropine, can lead to systemic toxicity. Overdosage of the less potent cycloplegics can have the same results.

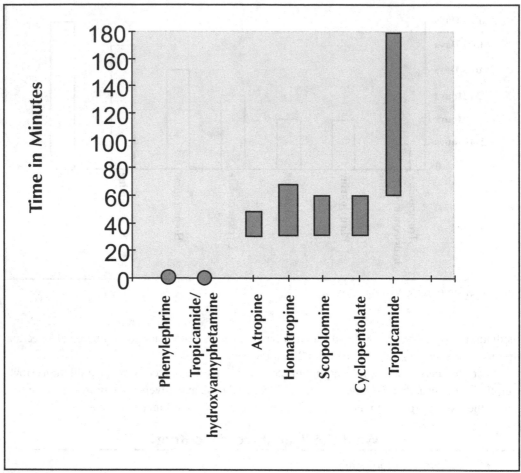

Figure 4-3. Time to maximum cycloplegia.

Systemic toxicity is hallmarked by flushing (reddening) of skin, dryness of skin and mouth, irregular and rapid pulse, hallucination, speech difficulty, and loss of coordination. Physicians, technicians, and parents should all be aware of these symptoms, especially when cycloplegics are given to children. Also, these drugs should be administered carefully to those with Down syndrome, who tend to have an increased response to these medications.

What the Patient Needs to Know

- Watch children, especially if premedicated, for signs of systemic toxicity: flushed skin, dryness of skin and mouth, irregular and rapid pulse, hallucinations, speech difficulty, loss of coordination.

Atropine

Atropine sulfate is available in 0.5%, 1%, 2%, and 3% solutions as well as 0.5% and 1% ophthalmic ointments. It is commonly used in the refraction of children and to treat severe

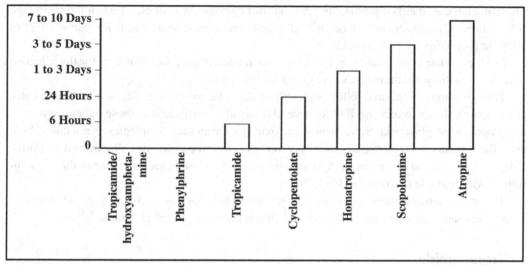

Figure 4-4. Time to cycloplegic recovery.

inflammatory conditions of the uveal tract. It is also used to blur the "good" eye as an alternative to patching in the treatment of amblyopia. The usual dosage for cycloplegic refraction in children is 1 drop twice daily for 1 to 3 days before the examination. The clinical usefulness of atropine must be weighed against its increased side effects and long duration, which can handicap the patient for many days after instillation. Though it is time tested and useful, there is a better choice for most situations.

Scopolamine

Scopolamine (Isopto-Hyoscine®) is available only as a 0.25% solution. Its main use is in the treatment of uveitis. It is rarely used for cycloplegic refraction. For uveitis, the recommended dosage is 1 drop 2 to 4 times daily; for refraction, the recommendation is 1 drop 1 hour before the examination.

Homatropine

Homatropine is available in 2% and 5% solutions. Its indications and dosages are the same as that of scopolamine. The major advantage it has over atropine and scopolamine is its decreased time of recovery. Though the mydriatic effect of homatropine is lengthy, its cycloplegic effect is much weaker. Therefore, homatropine is not the first drug of choice for fundus exam or cycloplegic refraction. Its main practical use is in the treatment of uveitis. The side effects of homatropine are the same as those for atropine (see above).

Cyclopentolate

Cyclopentolate (Cyclogyl®) is available as 0.5%, 1%, and 2% solutions. It is also marketed in 0.2% combined with 1% phenylephrine (Cyclomydril®). Cyclopentolate has many advantages over the previously mentioned cycloplegics. Its onset is faster (30 to 60 min), and recovery time is shorter (6 to 24 hours). Also, the time to peak mydriasis and cycloplegia are almost the same.

The clinician can, then, be reasonably sure that full cycloplegia is in effect when the pupils are fully dilated. Cyclopentolate is a better cycloplegic than homatropine and is similar in effect to atropine (but wears off more quickly).

Cyclopentolate is a versatile tool, not only for refractive purposes, but also for the effective relief of the ciliary inflammation seen in a variety of conditions.

Though stinging is normal following instillation, ocular hypersensitivity is rare. Cyclopentolate has been shown to increase IOP for several hours after instillation in those patients with primary open-angle glaucoma. Systemically, its toxicity mirrors the cycloplegics as a whole. However, there seems to be increased central nervous system effects such as hallucination and difficulty with speech and coordination. Systemic toxicity is more often seen with use of the 2% solution or with multiple drops of the 1% solution.

The recommended dosage for cycloplegic refraction is 2 drops given 5 min apart, 30 to 45 min before the examination. For uveitis, the 1% solution is commonly instilled 3 times daily.

Tropicamide

Tropicamide (Mydriacyl®) is the weakest-acting cycloplegic agent. For most situations, it lacks the clinical effectiveness and duration to be useful for its cycloplegic effects alone. Its popularity is due to the fact that it has the quickest onset and fastest recovery of mydriasis versus all other mydriatic and cycloplegic drugs. This makes tropicamide ideal for routine fundus evaluation from the standpoint of both the patient and physician.

Tropicamide is available in both 0.5% and 1% solutions. As mentioned previously, it is also available as a 0.25% solution in combination with 1% hydroxyamphetamine. Using phenylephrine or hydroxyamphetamine in combination with one of the cycloplegic drugs (usually tropicamide) has a synergistic effect. (A synergist is a drug that works in conjunction with another drug toward a common goal. The effects of both drugs are enhanced, giving a greater result than simple addition.) This works because the drugs each have a separate site of action. Thus, a larger pupil dilation can be obtained with the combination than when either agent is used alone. It is common practice to use 1 drop of 2.5% phenylephrine followed in 5 min by 1 drop of tropicamide when maximal pupil dilation is necessary (eg, when examining for retinal breaks).

Similar to other agents in its class, tropicamide also stings upon instillation and can raise IOP. However, the pressure rise is usually insignificant and short lasting, making tropicamide ideal for use in glaucoma patients.

Systemic reactions to tropicamide are extremely uncommon. The central nervous system and vascular reactions seen with the other cycloplegics have not been demonstrated in tropicamide. It is, thus, the safest agent to use for mydriasis in children and patients with diabetes or cardiovascular disease.

Ophthalmic Dyes

Ophthalmic dyes are valuable diagnostic aids. They enable the physician to better view the ocular surface and the retinal or choroidal vasculature.

Adverse effects are minimal when any ophthalmic dyes are administered topically to the eye. However, they readily stain skin, fingers, and clothes. Be careful when handling or administering them, and keep the amount used to a minimum.

Fluorescein Sodium

Fluorescein is a yellow or orange dye that appears bright green when viewed under cobalt blue light. There are many clinical uses for fluorescein dye. Administered topically, it can aid in the detection of corneal abrasions or foreign bodies. It is used when performing Goldmann applanation tonometry, evaluating the fit of rigid contact lenses, and studying the stability of the tear film. Fluorescein is also useful in evaluating for a wound leak following intraocular surgery. Injected or taken orally, it is invaluable for visualizing abnormalities in retinal circulation.

Topical Fluorescein

OptA
OptT
OphA
CL

When fluorescein is applied to the eye, the normal tear film will appear the same yellow color as the drop. Fluorescein does not penetrate the intact cornea. However, when the corneal surface is compromised or disrupted, as in the case of a corneal abrasion, the dye easily penetrates the cornea. When viewed through a cobalt blue filter, the abrasion glows bright green, highlighting the defect and making it easily visible. If the corneal defect is large enough, the fluorescein can actually penetrate into the anterior chamber, giving the appearance of green aqueous flare and obscuring proper evaluation.

Regular fluorescein dye must not be used in an eye wearing a soft contact lens. The dye may penetrate the matrix of the contact lens and cause permanent discoloration. The large molecular size of the fluorescein solution Fluorexon (Fluoresoft®) keeps the dye from penetrating the contact lens matrix. Fluorexon is, therefore, useful in evaluating the fit of both rigid and soft contact lenses. After instillation and assessment, the lenses should be removed, washed, and rinsed with saline. The lenses may appear slightly colored, but most of the dye will be removed with cleaning. Lenses with hydration greater than 55% pick up the most coloration and require the most rinsing. Any residual coloration will dissipate after the lenses are reinserted. Do not use peroxide-based cleaning solutions in conjunction with fluorexon, because peroxide can cause the dye to bond to the contact lens.

For topical diagnostic purposes, fluorescein sodium is available in 2% solution. The problem with fluorescein solution is that it can become easily contaminated with bacteria. Therefore, for specific use in applanation tonometry, 0.25% fluorescein is combined with a preservative and a local anesthetic, either 0.4% benoxinate (Fluress®) or 0.5% proparacaine HCl (Fluoracaine®). In combination, these solutions are very resistant to contamination and are popular for this reason as well as convenience. Fluorescein is also available in impregnated strips of filter paper (Fluretts®, Fluor-I-Strip®). These strips have the advantage of being less messy and are resistant to contamination. First, the strips are moistened with anesthetic or irrigating solution, releasing the dye. The moistened strip is then applied to the conjunctiva or cornea depending on the need.

Systemic Fluorescein

Fluorescein sodium is available in ampules of 10% and 25% solutions for injection and use in ophthalmic angiography. For angiography, the fluorescein is administered intravenously. Through direct visualization and photography, the dye is seen as it enters the blood vessels, enabling one to evaluate the integrity of the retinal vasculature. This procedure is critical to the diagnosis and localization of many different retinal abnormalities.

A similar alternative is oral fluorography. In this technique, fluorescein powder or a 10% solution is combined with a citrus drink over ice, which the patient drinks. After a period of time, the retina is viewed. This technique has less risk and fewer side effects compared to intravenous fluorescein and has gained many proponents over the years, especially in Europe.

However, using oral fluorography limits the conditions that may be viewed and has not gained widespread popularity.

Systemic use of fluorescein sodium is not without risk and adverse effects. Most commonly, the skin takes on a yellow or tannish discoloration that fades over a 36-hour period. The patient's urine will also turn bright yellow, and a strong aftertaste may develop. These effects are transient, but patients must be forewarned about them before administration. Nausea, headache, and upset stomach can also result. Hypersensitivity is rare but can develop, ranging from itching and hives to full-blown anaphylactic shock. If anaphylactic shock develops, immediate measures must be taken. Therefore, medical personnel must be present when systemic fluorescein is used. Appropriate medications and supplies (an antihistamine, 0.1% epinephrine, a soluble steroid, aminophylline IV, and oxygen) must be kept on hand to deal with this unlikely emergency.

What the Patient Needs to Know

- Soft contact lenses must not be worn until all fluorescein is gone from the eye. Otherwise, lenses may become discolored.

- After injection of sodium fluorescein, it is normal to have yellowish discoloration of skin and urine.

Rose Bengal

Rose bengal, as its name implies, is a red or rose colored dye. It specifically binds to mucus as well as to dead and devitalized tissue. It does not stain most epithelial defects and does not permeate the anterior chamber. Rose bengal is useful in the diagnosis of corneal and conjunctival damage secondary to ocular surface disease, such as dry eye and herpetic keratitis.

Rose bengal is available in a 1% solution and impregnated filter paper strips (Rosetts®). Patients may notice some stinging upon instillation, but other reactions are rare. The staining may persist for several hours after instillation. An important clinical note is that rose bengal staining should always be performed before fluorescein is introduced into the eye because the fluorescein can mask the appearance of rose bengal. Lastly, rose bengal has been shown to have mild antiviral properties. Therefore, if a viral culture is to be taken from the eye (admittedly a seldom done procedure), this must be done before instillation of rose bengal.

Indocyanine Green

Aside from specific uses in cataract and vitreoretinal surgery, the use of indocyanine green (ICG) is common in ophthalmic angiography. Due to its unique binding properties, it enables a better view of the choroidal vasculature, a structure that is often masked in traditional fluorescein angiography.

ICG is available in both powder (25 and 50 mg) and solution (10 and 40 mg single-use vials). The solution is unstable, however, and must be used within 10 hours. The powder must be dissolved only with the provided aqueous solvent.

ICG contains sodium iodine and must be used with caution in patients with iodine sensitivity. However, the likelihood of significant reaction is minimal; when used intravenously, toxic reactions are rare.

Trypan Blue

Trypan Blue has received the most recent United States Food and Drug Administration (FDA) approval for use as an ophthalmic dye. For years, cataract surgeons have looked for better ways of visualizing the lens capsule during cataract surgery. Usually relying on the retinal red reflex, observation becomes difficult in very dense or mature cataracts, and inability to view the capsule clearly increases the risk of surgery.

Trypan Blue 0.06% (Vision Blue® - Dutch Ophthalmic Research Center) aids in viewing the capsular opening (capsulorhexis) during cataract surgery. The solution is available in ready-to-use syringes and is injected into the anterior lens capsule at the time of surgery. Before the dye's arrival on the market, surgeons had to either have it formulated at a pharmacy (on a patient-by-patient basis) or use other agents, such as ICG or fluorescein dye (though none were FDA approved for such use). Approval aside, Vision Blue offers advantages over ICG in that it requires no mixing and provides better and longer intraoperative visualization.

The safety and effectiveness of Vision Blue has been established in pediatric patients. Adverse reactions are generally self-limited and of short duration. They include discoloration of intraocular lenses and staining of the posterior lens capsule and the vitreous.

Bibliography

Bartlett JD, ed. *Ophthalmic Drug Facts*. St. Louis, Mo: Wolters Kluwer Health; 2005.

Bartlett JD, Jannus SD. *Clinical Ocular Pharmacology*. 4th ed. Boston, Mass: Butterworth-Heinmann Publishing; 2001.

Melton, Thomas R. 4th Annual guide to therapeutic drugs. Norwalk, Conn: Optometric Management; 1995.

Onofrey BE. Clinical Optometric Pharmacology and Therapeutics. Philadelphia, Pa: JB Lippincott; 1992.

Physician's Desk Reference for Ophthalmology. 33rd ed. Montvale, NJ: Thomson PDR; published annually.

Webb J. FDA approves capsular dye to assist cataract surgery. *Ophthalmology Times*. 2005:30 (5).

Chapter 5

Use of Ocular Lubricants, Cyclosporine, and Osmotics

KEY POINTS

- Ocular lubricants are the initial therapeutic choice for ocular dryness. Preservative-free preparations should be used whenever possible.

- Topical hyperosmotics are used to decrease corneal edema resulting from a variety of conditions and are helpful in increasing vision and comfort.

- Mucomimetic, irrigating, and coupling solutions have valuable but limited roles in ophthalmic care.

- The space-occupying, protective, and inert nature of viscoelastics make them a critical component of intraocular surgery.

Topical Lubricants

Dry eye, including its associated symptoms, is the most common presenting condition in ophthalmic practice. It is caused by a deficiency in 1 of the 3 layers composing the tear film. Dry eye is a condition that can be exacerbated by concurrent eyelid conditions, arid and windy environments, and extended near work. It is more frequently found in the elderly, it appears in women more than men, and it is associated with a number of systemic and dermatologic conditions. Systemic medications (including hormone replacement, birth control pills, steroids, and diuretics) may lead to this condition. Presenting symptoms include a "gritty or sandy feeling," burning, and even paradoxical increased tearing. In any event, the standard first-line treatment is the use of tear supplementing artificial tear drops and lubricating ointments. The artificial tears and related ointments are designed to mimic the tears, substitute for the defective properties, and stabilize the existing tear film.

Due to their nature and makeup, artificial tears and lubricating ointments are free of any adverse effects, with the exception of transient blurring and preservative toxicity. Artificial tears and ointments should not be used with contact lenses in place. Only recommended rewetting and contact lens solutions should be used.

What the Patient Needs to Know

- Certain medications, such as antihistamines, birth control pills, hormone replacement, and diuretics, increase dryness.

    - If used more than 3 or 4 times daily, nonpreserved tears are recommended.

    - Temporary blurring may result after instillation of artificial tears, especially with the thicker drops.

    - If your eyes are dry, avoid using drops that "get the red out." These may make dryness worse.

    - Dry eye is a chronic condition. Artificial tears should be used regularly and frequently if therapy is to be helpful.

    - Tear drops should be used *before* the eyes start feeling dry and irritated.

    - Though it seems backwards, watery eyes can be the result of dryness. Use the drops as your doctor prescribes. They will help.

Artificial Tears

The number of artificial tear preparations available over the counter is overwhelming (Tables 5-1 and 5-2). This is evidenced by a single glance at the shelf in the local pharmacy. Artificial tears contain various components and different combinations of buffers, tonicity agents, polymers, and occasionally preservatives and vitamins.

The major therapeutic component in artificial tears is the water-soluble polymer. These agents determine the viscosity (thickness) of the artificial tear solution and aid in tear stabilization. They include methylcellulose, hydroxyethyl cellulose, hydroxypropyl cellulose, hydroxypropyl methylcellulose, carboxymethylcellulose, and polyvinyl alcohol. Electrolytes help to maintain pH and tonicity of the solution. Examples of pH buffers include boric acid, sodium bicarbonate, sodium borate, hydrochloric acid, sodium citrate, sodium hydroxide, and sodium prosphate. Tonicity agents include dextran, dextrose, potassium chloride, propylene glycol, and sodium chloride.

Table 5-1
Partial List of Nonpreserved Artificial Tears (Brand Names)

Bion Tears
Celluvisc
Hypotears PF
Refresh Plus
Refresh Endura
Tears Naturale Free
Theratears

Table 5-2
Selected Preserved Artificial Tears (Brand Names)

AKWA Tears
Aquasite
Computer Eye Drops
Genteal
Hypotears
Moisture Eyes
Nutra-Tears
Rhoto Zi
Systane
Tears Naturale Forte
Viva Drops
Visine Tears

Preservatives are included in multi-dose preparations of artificial tears, decreasing the risk of bacterial contamination. Benzalkonium chloride, EDTA, and Polyquaternium-1 are some of the common preservatives used in artificial tear preparations. Due to the likelihood of developing a preservative-related toxicity, solutions with preservatives must be used with some precautions, if used on a frequent basis.

There are a few artificial tear preparations with added vitamins and antioxidants. For example, Viva Drops® add vitamin A to their preparation while Nutratear® contains vitamin B12. Some studies suggest that vitamin supplementation is of benefit in treating severe dry eye and other forms of keratitis, including superior limbal keratoconjunctivitis. Theratears® has a patented electrolyte balance that exactly matches that of natural human tears. This formulation may prove to have additional benefits to the corneal and conjunctival health of the dry eye patient.

The frequency of administration is dependent upon the severity of the condition. The drops may be instilled as infrequently as once or twice daily or as often as every hour, as necessary. To prevent preservative toxicity, it is recommended that nonpreserved artificial tear solutions be used if drops are prescribed for more than 3 or 4 times daily use. Nonpreserved artificial tears, however, are not as convenient due to their single-dose containers and increased expense.

Table 5-3
Selected Lubricating Agents in Order of Increasing Viscosity (Brand Names)
Hypotears
Refresh
Tears Plus
Tears Naturale
Bion Tears
Ocucoat
Celluvisc

Adapted from data obtained from Storz Ophthalmics, St. Louis, Mo.

A beneficial development has been the introduction of the "disappearing" preservatives in artificial tear solutions. On contacting the eye, the preservative is converted to dilute hydrogen peroxide, which then changes into water and oxygen within a minute of contacting the eye. The cornea is much less likely to develop preservative toxicity with this short contact time. The advantage is the benefits of nonpreserved tears with the convenience, safety, and value of a preserved solution. Commercially available products such as Genteal® have been a welcome addition to the artificial tear market.

Viscosity is another property of artificial tears that must be considered. Viscosity varies among the various tear preparations available (Table 5-3). More viscous solutions promote longer contact time and increased therapeutic benefits. The disadvantage of viscous tear solutions is their tendency to blur vision temporarily; the more viscous the solution, the more blurred the vision.

Clinicians have developed elaborate programs to determine the appropriate viscosity for a given patient and condition. These programs are usually some sort of subjective single-elimination tournament with the winner determined after a period of up to 6 weeks. Patients may get frustrated with the length, expense, and time involved in the program. It may be best to give the patient a set frequency and send him or her home with multiple samples of varying viscosity. The patient should then find the tear he or she prefers and use it. The patient might also be given information regarding the pros and cons of the different drops based on their makeup, viscosity, and cost.

In addition to administration by drops, there have been a few products introduced that deliver the solution as a spray mist. Though these products have gained a following by some patients, they have not yet achieved widespread popularity by patients or physicians in the therapeutic treatment of dry eye.

The extraocular use of viscoadherent and viscoelastic agents in the treatment of dry eye has also been advocated. Marketed under the name Ocucoat®, hydroxypropyl methylcellulose is available as a viscous artificial tear. Also, sodium hyaluronate has been applauded by some clinicians for its ability to promote tear film stability, although it is not available as an artificial tear preparation at the time of this publication.

There are varying clinical opinions on the best agent and program in treating dry eye with artificial tears. Patients often get confused and frustrated with the many options, chronic and frequent drop use, expense, and inconvenience. These aspects should be discussed with the patient at the office visit to ensure proper compliance and, ultimately, successful treatment of the condition.

Lastly, many patients often use ocular decongestants to soothe dry eyes. These drops "get the red out" but have minimal contact time with the eye, provide little lubrication, and can actually

Table 5-4
Selected Ophthalmic Lubricating Ointments (Brand Names)
Preserved
AKWA Tears Ointment
Hypotears Ointment
Lacri-lube SOP
Refresh PM
Tears Renewed

make the eye more red and dry, if used frequently. Inform all dry eye patients that they should stay away from these drops. These ocular decongestants do have a place (as will be discussed in the upcoming chapter), but that place is not in the treatment of dry eye.

There has been some research and clinical study looking at the use of viscoelastic agents extraocularly in the treatment of dry eye. Marketed under the name Ocucoat®, hydroxymethyl-cellulose is now available as a viscous artificial tear. Sodium hyaluronate has been applauded by some for its ability to promote tear film stability, but not all agree with this assessment.

Ophthalmic Lubricating Ointments

Ophthalmic lubricating ointments are similar to artificial tears in their makeup. In addition, ointments contain emollients such as petrolatum, mineral oil, and lanolin. Applied as a small ribbon to the inferior cul-de-sac, these products dissolve at ocular surface temperature, spread with the tear film, and lubricate and protect the tissues. The increased contact time and viscosity of ophthalmic lubricating ointments make them very useful in the treatment of severe dry eye or in cases of exposure secondary to nocturnal lagophthalmos (a condition where the lids do not entirely close during sleep). Though ointments have advantages, their major drawback, like all ophthalmic ointments, is the transient blurring of vision. Ointments are, thus, used primarily at night, unless the dry eye is significant enough to warrant otherwise. A list of selected lubricating ointments is provided in Table 5-4.

Sometimes, a patient will use a viscous artificial tear preparation such as Celluvisc® for nighttime use rather than an ointment. These viscous solutions do not have the prolonged contact time or lengthy staying power necessary for nighttime use.

Sustained-Release Lubrication

Lastly, there is a solid sustained-release tear product available. Marketed as Lacrisert®, it is a preservative-free pellet containing 5 mg of hydropropyl cellulose. When placed in the inferior cul-de-sac, the pellet swells and releases its polymer into the tear film for up to 24 hours. This sustained-release action can be beneficial in the most severe cases of dry eye. However, disadvantages such as cost, patient intolerance, and excessive blurred vision have eliminated this product as a front-line weapon in the battle against dry eye.

Topical Cyclosporine

For many years, clinicians have valued the immunosuppressive effects of cyclosporine in the management of moderate to severe dry eye. Originally, however, it was used off-label and had to be formulated by a pharmacy. Topical steroids have also proved beneficial but have a lower safety profile for long-term use, with risks such as cataract formation and increased IOP. However, with the introduction of Restasis® (Allergan), there is now a readily available, effective alternative to artificial tears and punctual occlusion in the management of dry eye. Restasis is the first commercially available ophthalmic cyclosporine drop.

Restasis is a nonpreserved 0.05% cyclosporine solution that is dosed twice daily. It is important to note that in most patients, it takes 4 to 8 weeks (and sometimes longer) to achieve a meaningful effect, and (like artificial tears) the treatment can be chronic. Restasis is not inexpensive, and for some, the cost can be a factor with continuing compliance. Restasis therapy has proven effective long-term in patients where artificial tear therapy alone has been ineffective.

What the Patient Needs to Know

- Restasis works to increase tear production by reducing inflammation.

- It may take 1 to 3 months for significant improvement to be noted with the use of Restasis. Stay the course.

- The medication may sting.

- You may continue to use regular tear drops as needed.

Artificial Eye Lubricant/Cleaning Agents

Benzalkonium chloride 0.02% and tyloxapol 0.25% are commercially available as a combination solution marketed under the name Enuclene®. It is used to clean and lubricate prosthetic eyes. The benzalkonium chloride is an antibacterial agent that acts to disinfect the artificial eye and socket. Tyloxapol is a detergent that liquifies the solid matter that accumulates on the prosthesis.

Enuclene is applied just as one would apply any topical ocular solution, with a normal frequency of 1 drop 4 times daily. Occasionally, the prosthetic eye may be removed and cleaned with this solution. In this case, one would apply several drops to the artificial eye and then rinse with saline. A drop or 2 is then applied before reinsertion.

Contact Lens Coupling Solutions

Hydroxypropyl methylcellulose 2.5% (Gonak®, Goniosol®) and hydroxyethyl cellulose (Gonioscopic Prism Solution®) are used as coupling agents when gonioscopy or contact fundoscopy are performed. These solutions create a cushion between the lens and the cornea and provide the optical continuity necessary for visualization with these lenses. Because optical continuity is the goal, bubbles in the solution should be avoided. The bottle should not be shaken. Store the bottle upside down when not in use so that any bubbles will rise up and away from the dropper tip.

The major drawback with these solutions is that they may cause keratitis and decreased corneal clarity after removal of the lens. The patient's eye will be mildly red, irritated, and sticky

Table 5-5
Selected Extraocular Irrigating Solutions (Brand Names)

AK-Rinse
Blinx
Collyrium Fresh Eyes
Dacriose
Eye Stream
Eye Wash

after the use of viscous coupling solutions. Some physicians advocate irrigating the remaining solution from the eye after the exam is complete.

In an attempt to eliminate the drawbacks of these coupling agents, many practitioners have substituted a viscous rigid contact lens solution like Soac-lens® or a viscous artificial tear solution like Celluvisc®. These solutions allow better visualization through the cornea after their use and cause less corneal irritation and patient discomfort. The disadvantages of these less viscous solutions are their decreased corneal adherence and propensity for bubble formation.

Intraocular Irrigating Solutions

`Srg`

Intraocular irrigating solutions have no pharmacologic action. Their sole purpose is to irrigate the intraocular tissues during surgery and to provide the metabolites necessary to maintain cellular function. Historically, sterile saline and ringer's lactate were used as irrigating solutions. These proved inadequate due to endothelial cell breakdown. This led to the changes in formulation of today's intraocular irrigating solutions.

Intraocular irrigating solutions must have the same tonicity as the ocular tissues—pH must remain at 7.4; a pH below 7 or above 8 has been shown to cause cell death after prolonged exposure. The solutions are marketed under several names including Balanced Salt Solution, BSS, and Endosol®. All contain sodium chloride, potassium chloride, magnesium chloride, sodium acetate, sodium citrate, and sodium hydroxide or hydrochloric acid in specific concentrations. As a result of their nature, intraocular irrigating solutions are free of preservatives. Given this and their nonpharmacologic properties, adverse effects and allergies are extremely rare.

All commercially available intraocular irrigating solutions work well for use during shorter surgical procedures. For surgery lasting longer than 1 hour, a more advanced preparation is recommended. Available in solutions such as BSS Plus®, they contain added nutrients to promote greater tissue health during longer surgeries. BSS Plus is packaged as 2 separate components that must be mixed before surgery. Once mixed, the solution remains stable for only 24 hours.

Extraocular Irrigating Solutions

`OptA`
`OptT`
`OphA`
`Srg`

Just like their intraocular counterparts, extraocular irrigating solutions exhibit no pharmacologic action. They are also isotonic and pH balanced. They are available over the counter without prescription and under many names (Table 5-5). They have a variety of uses both in and out of the office. Extraocular irrigating solution is used for foreign body removal, general cleaning, nasolacrimal irrigation, and removal of coupling solutions after gonioscopy and similar procedures.

Administration is accomplished through a direct stream from the bottle or with an eye cup. The eye cup should be filled halfway with irrigating solution then applied tightly to the eye. With the eyes open wide, the patient tilts his or her head backward. The eye should be rotated and blinked several times. The solution is then discarded.

Extraocular solutions contain preservatives, and epithelial toxicity can occur with chronic use. They should never be used as a substitute for saline solution when storing or rinsing contact lenses because they may increase the likelihood of developing a severe sight-threatening infection.

What the Patient Needs to Know

- Irrigation is not a substitute for artificial tears.
    - Irrigation solution is not for rinsing or storing contact lenses.
    - If your symptoms persist after irrigating the eye, professional care should be sought.
    - A qualified eyecare professional should be seen after any chemical splashes in the eye, even after rinsing.

Mucolytics

Acetylcystine is a mucolytic agent used infrequently in ophthalmic practice. A mucolytic agent is an agent that breaks down mucus and reduces viscosity. It is commonly used in bronchopulmonary conditions. Acetylcystine is not approved by the FDA for ocular use. Nonetheless, it can be valuable for treating conditions like filamentary keratitis and associated recurrent corneal erosion where excess mucus formation is present.

Acetylcystine is available for bronchial and pulmonary conditions as Mucomyst® in 10% and 20% solutions. Ocularly, it can be used as 10% solution but is more commonly diluted to 2% or 5%. It may be diluted by mixing with artificial tears or saline and then placed into a dropper bottle. These diluted solutions are not preserved and should be refrigerated after preparation. They should be kept no longer than 14 days. Due to its chemical makeup, acetylcystine emits a foul odor like rotten eggs. This should not be confused with spoilage or contamination.

What the Patient Needs to Know

- Acetylcystine should be kept refrigerated.
- The solution smells like rotten eggs. This does not mean the drug has spoiled!
- Discard any left over solution after 14 days.

Srg

Viscoelastic Agents

Viscoelastic agents are tissue-protective and space-occupying substances. They are primarily used during surgical procedures such as intraocular lens implantation and keratoplasty. For instance, viscoelastics help to maintain both a deep anterior chamber and capsular bag during cataract surgery. They also coat and protect fragile endothelial cells from the friction and trauma of intraocular surgery.

Table 5-6
Viscoelastics (Brand Names)
Biolon
Duovisc
Healon
Healon GV
Healon 5
Ocucoat
Provisc
Viscoat
Vitrax

There are currently multiple viscoelastic agents available on the market for use during anterior segment surgery (Table 5-6). All products, except Ocucoat®, have sodium hyaluronate as their major viscoelastic component. Ocucoat uses hydroxypropyl methylcellulose instead.

The products differ slightly in their qualities. The differences are in their viscosity, elasticity, ability to coat and protect the endothelial cells and ocular tissues, as well as others. The optimal viscoelastic varies depending on the surgeon, specific need, and intended use.

Adverse reactions to viscoelastics are very uncommon due to their relatively inert nature. They do not interfere with wound healing and are designed not to initiate an inflammatory reaction within the eye. There are concerns by some that hydroxypropyl methylcellulose (which, unlike sodium hyaluronate, is not physiologic) may increase the risk of adverse reactions. These concerns have not been justified clinically, however. Lastly, viscoelastics may cause an increase in IOP when left in the eye after surgery.

What the Patient Needs to Know

- These drops sting!
- It is often advisable to put drops in more frequently upon waking in the morning.

Topical Hyperosmotics

OphT

Osmotic agents have multiple uses in ophthalmic practice. Used systemically, they can help to reduce IOP in glaucoma management. Topical hyperosmotics are useful in reducing corneal swelling caused by fluid retention. This swelling is known as corneal edema and can result from a variety of conditions.

The cornea is a 5-layered structure. Its 3 major tissue layers are the endothelium, the stroma, and the epithelium. The endothelium is the innermost tissue of the cornea and is bathed posteriorly by the aqueous humor. The stroma is the middle, making up about 90% of the thickness of the cornea. It is composed of tightly packed collagen fibers, which maintain the structure and clarity of the cornea. The epithelium is the outermost surface of the cornea, acting as a barrier against external forces. It is bathed by the tear film. These 3 components work together to keep the cornea relatively dehydrated at 78% hydration, which maintains maximum clarity. The cornea is capable of swelling to approximately 98% hydration, which is close to the state maintained by the adjacent sclera.

To maintain the state of dehydration, the endothelium prevents excess movement of water into the cornea from the aqueous. The epithelium prevents the uptake of water from the tear film. Under normal situations, this system works remarkably well. However, changes in the structure of these tissues, particularly the endothelium, can change the equilibrium. Trauma, corneal dystrophy, or other pathology can cause a breakdown of the barriers, causing the cornea to become swollen or edematous. A sudden increase in IOP, as seen in acute angle-closure glaucoma, can also force fluid into the cornea. No matter what the cause of the edema, the collagen matrix of the stroma becomes disrupted, and epithelial clouding occurs, leading to reduced vision.

How do topical hyperosmotics work? First, water moves by means of osmosis. This means that water will move across a membrane from a dilute solution to a more concentrated one. A topical hypertonic solution is more concentrated than the ocular tissue, and, therefore, water moves toward it, across the epithelium, and out of the cornea. The result is less corneal edema, greater patient comfort, and improved vision. These solutions do have their limitations, as they tend to work best when the edema is located in the epithelium. They are less effective against edema deeper in the corneal stroma. The 2 topical hyperosmotics that are routinely used in ophthalmic practice are sodium chloride and glycerin.

Sodium Chloride

As mentioned in Chapter 1, the corneal tear film is equivalent in tonicity to a 0.9% sodium chloride solution. For use as a topical hyperosmotic, sodium chloride is available as 2% and 5% solutions and a 5% ointment (Muro-128®, Ak-Nacl®, and Adsorbonac®). The 5% solution has been shown to be most clinically useful in improving both patient comfort and vision in cases of mild to moderate epithelial edema. The usual regimen is application of 1 drop 4 times daily and ointment applied at bedtime. However, it is often advisable to direct the patient to administer 1 drop each hour for the first few hours after waking, when corneal edema is usually worse.

Topical sodium chloride is nontoxic, and allergic reactions are uncommon. However, these preparations do sting upon instillation, and the patient needs to be forewarned.

Glycerin/Glycerol

Glycerin is another osmotic solution. Glycerin absorbs water when the 2 are placed in contact with one another and, thus, exerts a hypertonic effect. When glycerin is administered topically to an edematous epithelium, it temporarily clears the edema and its associated corneal haze. The hypertonic effect of glycerin is transient, with its peak effect around 2 minutes. Topical glycerin is painful when applied, so it is advisable to use a topical anesthetic before instillation. Due to its painful nature and its short activity, it is not useful for chronic therapy. However, it is extremely useful to clear epithelial edema to allow visualization when performing gonioscopy or ophthalmoscopy in the office. This is often necessary in patients with acute angle-closure glaucoma. Other than painful stinging, adverse effects to topically applied glycerin are rare.

Bibliography

Bartlett J. Artificial tears and ointments for treatment of dry eye. *EyeCare Technology Magazine*. 1995; 5(3):25-27.

Bartlett JD, ed. *Ophthalmic Drug Facts*. St. Louis, Mo: Wolters Kluwer Health; 2005.

Bartlett JD, Jaanus SD, eds. *Clinical Ocular Pharmacology*. 4th ed. Boston, Mass: Butterworth Heinmann Publishing; 2001.

Friedlander M, Bartlett J. Biotechnology: Getting a handle on dry eyes. *EyeCare Technology Magazine*. 1996; 6(5):33,41,50.

Kanski JJ. *Clinical Ophthalmology*. 2nd ed. Boston, Mass: Butterworths; 1989.

Kauffman PL, Alm A. *Adler's Physiology of the Eye*. 10th ed. St. Louis, Mo: Mosby; 2003.

Melton R, Thomas R. 2004 Clinical Guide to Ophthalmic Drugs. *Review of Optometry*. August 15, 2004 (suppl): 8a-12a.

Melton R, Thomas R. *4th Annual Guide to Therapeutic Drugs*. Norwalk, Conn: Optometric Management; 1995.

Morrill KX, Snow M. Understanding viscoelastics: Think motor oil. *Review of Ophthalmology*. 1995; 2(2):65-68.

Onefrey BE, ed. *Clinical Optometric Pharmacology and Therapeutics*. Philadelphia, Pa: JB Lippincott; Williams & Wilkins, 1991.

Physician's Desk Reference. 59th ed. (33rd edition for ophthalmology, 26th edition for nonprescription drugs) Montvale, NJ: Thomson PDR; published annually.

Wilson ED. New dry-eye drops have vanishing preservative. *Primary Care Optometry News*. 1996; 1(3):34.

Chapter 6

Vasoconstrictors, Antihistamines, and Mast Cell Stabilizers

KEY POINTS

- Ocular antihistamine and decongestant combinations have some value in treating mild allergic conjunctivitis. They are inexpensive and easily obtained over the counter (OTC). However, they are often ineffective.

- Any product containing a decongestant should be used sparingly. Frequent use can result in increased redness and dryness.

- Mast cell stabilizers are useful in treating chronic ocular allergic symptoms. Preventative in nature, they must be used religiously, and their effect is often noticed only after days of treatment.

The Allergic Reaction

An allergic reaction is simply the overresponse of the immune system to a specific stimulus, usually environmental. This stimulus is called an antigen. There are 4 basic types of allergic reactions. We are all very familiar with the type 1 response. This reaction is seen as a result of hay fever, bee stings, cats, dogs, or even medications. It is the cause of the itchy, watery eyes, and runny nose many of us experience each spring when we cut the grass or stroll through the park. A brief look at the cause of this response will help us better understand the treatment of these conditions.

The allergic process begins when the body first comes in contact with an antigen, pollen for example (Figure 6-1). The body then produces cells, called antibodies, to target this specific antigen. The next time the body comes in contact with the pollen, these antibodies are activated. The antibodies attach to certain cells, called mast cells, and the process of degranulization begins. When a mast cell degranulates, many substances are released. One of these substances is called histamine. Histamine and other biochemicals spread throughout the body, including the eye. Certain receptors await the arrival of histamine. When the histamine attaches to a receptor (like a key fits a lock), swelling, tearing, redness, and itching result.

The best solution to the allergy problem is to stop the cycle. The most successful way to do this is to simply eliminate the cause, or antigen. Most of the time, however, it is very hard to identify the antigen, and even if we can, we cannot avoid it. Tear supplements, such as artificial tears, are useful in allergic conjunctivitis because they help to flush the antigen away from the ocular surface. Cold compresses help to decrease swelling and slow the immune response.

What the Patient Needs to Know

- The best way to eliminate allergies is to avoid the cause—not always an easy task.
- Cold compresses can help to relieve symptoms of allergies.

Medically, mild to moderate allergies are handled at 3 different levels. At the lowest level, ocular decongestants constrict the superficial blood vessels and decrease associated redness. Further up the allergic response, antihistamines can be used to block histamine receptors and reduce the resulting symptoms. Antihistamines are not always effective because other biochemicals also cause allergic symptoms. Lastly, drugs called mast cell stabilizers prevent the initial process of degranulation from occurring. In this chapter, we will look at drugs from each of these levels.

Ocular Decongestants

Ocular decongestants, or vasoconstrictors, are useful in decreasing the redness and irritation of mild allergies. When administered topically, they constrict the superficial conjunctival blood vessels and, thus, reduce congestion and redness. These agents have no effect on the deeper episcleral vessels. Vasoconstriction occurs within minutes after administration of these drugs. There are currently 4 ocular decongestants available for use in cases of allergic conjunctivitis: phenylephrine, naphazoline, oxymetazoline, and tetrahydrozoline. All are available without prescription either alone or in combination with other agents (Tables 6-1 and 6-2).

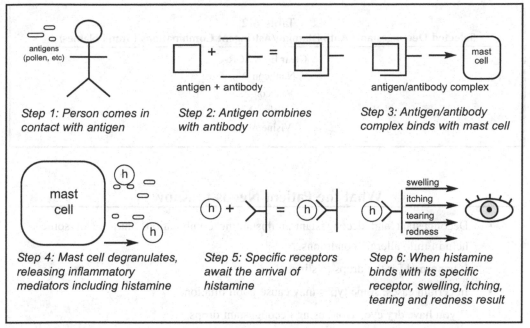

Figure 6-1. Pathway of typical histamine involved allergic response.

Table 6-1
Selected Decongestants (Brand Names)

Naphazoline
AK-Con (0.1%)
Albalon (0.1%)
All Clear (0.012%)
All Clear AR (0.03%)
Clear Eyes (0.012%)

Oxymetazoline
Visine LR (0.025%)

Phenylephrine
AK-Nefrin (0.12%)

Tetrahydrozoline
Eyesine (0.05%)
Murine Tears Plus (0.05%)
Visine (0.05%)
Visine Advanced Relief (0.05%)

Phenylephrine is available in a concentration of 0.12%. Though a strong mydriatic at a higher concentration, no mydriasis occurs at this lower strength if the cornea is intact. Phenylephrine has the shortest duration of all the ocular decongestants: about 30 to 90 minutes. The major drawback to phenylephrine is that it has been shown to cause rebound vessel dilation, a condition where the eyes may actually appear more red after use.

Table 6-2
Selected Decongestant/ Antihistamine/Astringent Combinations (Brand Names)
Clear Eyes ACR
Naphcon-A
Vasocon-A
Visine-A
Visine AC

What the Patient Needs to Know

- Decongestant and decongestant-antihistamine combinations may be of some help in mild allergic conditions.
- It is normal for the drops to sting.
- In certain cases, some types may cause pupil dilation.
- If you have dry eye, avoid using decongestant drops.
- If symptoms persist, see your eye doctor.

Naphazoline, oxymetazoline, and tetrahydrozoline are close relatives and, thus, have about the same effect. Naphazoline is found in concentrations of 0.1%, 0.012% and 0.03%. Clinical studies have shown lower concentrations to be as effective as larger ones. Oxymetazoline 0.025% and tetrahydrozoline 0.05% are also available in a variety of over-the-counter (OTC) solutions.

Ocular decongestants are relatively safe, though they should be used cautiously in children and those with vascular disorders. The major ocular side effect is transient stinging. Phenylephrine and naphazoline can cause mild pupillary dilation in patients with compromised corneas. Both may also cause a slight increase in IOP, as can tetrahydrozoline. Oxymetazoline does not seem to have this effect. The usual frequency for instilling these medications is 1 drop every 2 to 4 hours. Increasing the frequency is more effective than increasing the dosage.

Patients must be warned that prolonged symptoms can signal more serious eye disease. Though these agents can be helpful in a few situations, if symptoms persist, patients should seek care from qualified eyecare professionals.

Antihistamines

Oral Antihistamines

Orally administered antihistamines can be beneficial for patients with moderate to severe allergic conjunctivitis, rhinitis, and sinusitis. There are many products available both OTC and by prescription. The most common OTC oral antihistamines are diphenhydramine (ie, Benadryl®)

and chlorpheniramine (ie, Chlor-Trimeton®). Antihistamines generally have the same mechanism of action but differ in their potency and side effects.

Drowsiness is a major side effect of many antihistamines, and the development of products to minimize these effects has been successful and well received. As their tolerability has increased, so has their use in the treatment of ocular allergy. Due to their nondrowsy nature, Claritin® (also available OTC), Allegra®, Zyrtec®, and Clarinex® are the most commonly recommended in eyecare. *(Note to reader: Due to their high incidence of side effects and drug interactions, astemizol [ie, Hismanal®] and terfenadine [ie, Seldane®] were removed from the market).*

When used in the recommended dosage, oral antihistamines are generally safe and effective. However, anticholinergic effects like dry eye, dry mouth, and constipation can be common. Headaches also result occasionally. Allergies to antihistamines are uncommon but have been reported, more frequently with topical preparations. Lastly, patients taking certain antidepressants should not use these products due to the rare chance of developing severe hypertensive crisis.

What the Patient Needs to Know

- Oral antihistamines may cause drowsiness. Use caution when driving or operating machinery.

- Oral antihistamines can interact with certain medications. Check with your physician before taking.

- Other common side effects include dry eye, dry mouth, constipation, and headache.

Topical Antihistamines

When histamine binds to certain receptors, the allergic symptoms of redness, itching, tearing, and swelling result. Antihistamines block the histamine from binding and, thus, prevent some of these symptoms. It is important to realize that antihistamines do not stop the allergic response; they only block some of the acute symptoms. Topical antihistamines are available alone or in combination with ocular decongestants. They can be used by themselves or in conjunction with systemic antihistamines for cases of mild to moderate allergic conjunctivitis.

There are only 2 pure topical antihistamines available commercially: levocabastine 0.05% (Livostin®) and emadastine difumarate 0.05% (Emadine®). All other topical antihistamines are found in combination formulations. Unlike their inferior counterparts, Livostin and Emadine are powerful histamine blockers and are much more useful than the other antihistamines in treating the symptoms of allergic conjunctivitis. They may also be helpful for some patients in treating cases of myokymia (an involuntary twitch of the orbicularis muscle).

Though far more effective, Livostin and Emadine are more expensive than the other types They are normally prescribed for 4 to 6 times daily use. Aside from transient stinging, there are relatively few side effects.

Combination Therapy

Three other antihistamines are available for topical use in the eye. They are pyrilamine maleate, phemiramine maleate, and antizoline phosphate. All 3 are available OTC in combination with an ocular decongestant (see Table 6-2). Studies have shown that these antihistamine-decongestant combinations are more effective in relieving symptoms than their individual agents alone.

They are indicated for the relief of symptoms due to mild allergies. Their effect may be minimal (as with all antihistamines) because not all of the allergic response is due to histamine. Unlike Livostin and Emadine, these combination products are weak acting. The FDA has reviewed these solutions and listed them as "possibly effective." Though their therapeutic value is questionable, clinical relief is obtained by some patients. The main advantages these solutions have is that they are available OTC and are inexpensive. Topically, mild stinging is the only adverse effect normally encountered. Adverse systemic side effects can occur if systemic absorption is excessive. Patients with diabetes, hypertension, or cerebrovascular disease should use these products with caution. Finally, some of the commercially available products contain sulfites. These sulfites can cause allergic reactions in susceptible patients, who should avoid using them.

Astringents also act to reduce redness and irritation (see Table 6-2). Zinc and boric acid are examples of astringents. Some homeopathic products (Similasan®, Estivin II®) use solutions of rose petals and other natural substances to obtain this same effect. Although their effectiveness is often questioned, there is a small but loyal core of patients who swear by these products where all other therapeutic interventions have failed.

Mast Cell Stabilizers

Mast cells are located throughout the body, particularly the skin, respiratory tract, and conjunctiva. When a specific antigen causes mast cells to degranulate, a cascade of allergic events begins, resulting in the common allergic symptoms. Certain drugs, called mast cell stabilizers, prevent this degranulation and halt the resultant symptoms. They are very effective when used to minimize recurrence in the chronic treatment of ocular allergy.

Mast cell stabilizers contain no direct-acting antihistamine or decongestant. As a result, they do not give rapid relief to allergic symptoms. Once histamine and other allergic mediators have been released, mast cell stabilizers have no effect on the acute attack. Thus, it is best to begin using these medications prophylactically, before symptoms begin. If taken once symptoms have begun, several days may pass before improvement is noticed. Often, mast cell stabilizers are used in conjunction with another agent, like Livostin, during the acute phase of an allergic attack.

Currently, there are several mast cell stabilizers being marketed. First generation products include lodoxamide (Alomide®) and cromylyn sodium 4% (Crolom®, Opticrom®). Second generation products are pemirolast potassium 0.1% (Alamast®) and nedocromil sodium 2% (Alocril®). Usual administration is 4 to 6 times daily. A trial period of 3 weeks is advisable to determine the effectiveness of these drugs. Due to their delay in response to treatment, patients are often prescribed other medications to manage the acute symptoms during the initial stages of treatment. Like other topical antiallergy medications, they sting upon instillation. Otherwise, no ocular or systemic adverse effects occur. Mast cell stabilizers are also used in the treatment of other various ocular allergic conditions, such as vernal conjunctivitis and giant papillary conjunctivitis. They should not be used with contact lenses in place.

What the Patient Needs to Know

- Mast cell stabilizers do not help relieve acute allergic attacks.

- These drugs work best if treatment is begun prophylactically, before symptoms are noticed.

- Use for at least 3 weeks before deciding whether or not it helps.

- These drops usually sting.

- Do not use when wearing your contact lenses.

- Alocril® has a yellowish color. This is normal and does not mean the drop has gone bad.

Combined Properties

As mentioned, antihistamines are functional in treating some of the acute symptoms of allergic attack. Mast cell stabilizers are most useful in treating chronic and recurrent episodes, but they do not treat the acute symptoms that patients most often present. Both have their benefits, but researchers understood the need to incorporate the advantages of each in a single drop. Plopatadine HCL 0.1% and 0.2% (Patanol®) was the first drop on the market to give us this combination. Patanol works prophylacticly by coating the mast cells and preventing the degranulation and associated allergic flare-ups, and it works by quelling the acute itching by blocking the H1 histamine receptors. Dosed twice daily at the 0.1% strength and once daily at 0.2%, it not only is convenient for patients (increasing compliance) but highly effective at twice daily dosing.

The introduction of Patanol has since spawned other medications with a similar action: ketotifen fumarate 0.025% (Zaditor®), azelastine hydrochloride 0.05% (Optivar®), and epinastine hydrochloride 0.05% (Elestat®). These drugs appear to have clinical effectiveness for up to 8 hours. Contact lens wearers can instill these drops prior to lens insertion and again after they take the lenses out. On the down side, 4-time-a-day medications require that contacts be removed during the day for drop instillation.

Though the average cost of these drugs is higher than that of the antihistamines and mast cell stabilizers alone, the increased convenience, effectiveness, and single-drop dosing often make them a better value. Though normally supplied in 5-ml bottles, it is important to know (when comparing prices) that Optivar comes in 3-ml and 6-ml sizes. Another advantage is that these agents are approved for pediatric patients 3 years and older.

Bibliography

Bartlett JD, ed. *Ophthalmic Drug Facts*. St. Louis, Mo: Wolters Kluwer Health, 2005.

Bartlett JD, Jaanus SD. *Clinical Ocular Pharmacology*. 4th ed. Boston, Mass: Butterworth-Heinmann Publishing; 2001.

Care of the Patient with Conjunctivitis: An Optometric Clinical Practice Guideline (Pamphlet). St. Louis, Mo: American Optometric Assoc; 1995.

Marielo EN. *Human Anatomy and Physiology*. Redwood City, Calif: Benjamin/Cummings Publishing; 1989.

Melton R, Thomas R. *4th Annual Guide to Therapeutic Drugs*. Norwalk, Conn: Optometric Management; 1995.

Onefrey BE, ed. *Clinical Optometric Pharmacology and Therapeutics*. Philadelphia, Pa: JB Lippincott, Williams, & Wilkins; 1991.

Physicians' Desk Reference. 59th ed. (33rd edition for ophthalmology, 26th edition for nonprescription drugs) Montvale, NJ: Thomson PDR; published annually.

Shenan PW. A practical guide to allergy medications. *Review of Ophthalmology*. 1996; 3(3):112-117.

Silverman HM, ed. *The Pill Book*. 6th ed. New York, NY: Bantam Books; 1994.

Sowka JW, Gurwood AS, Kabat AG. *Handbook of Ocular Disease Management*. 6th ed. Review of Optometry. 2004 (suppl): 17a-21a.

Wilson ED. New dry-eye drops have vanishing preservative. *Primary Care Optometry News*. 1996; 1(3):34.

The Corticosteroids

- Corticosteroids are very potent inhibitors of inflammation but can cause serious side effects.

- Patients on corticosteroid therapy must be monitored closely. Long-term, chronic use of these drugs is not advised.

- Topical corticosteroids rarely cause adverse systemic effects.

- Ocular effects such as elevated IOP, posterior subcapsular cataract, and herpes keratitis activation can occur frequently.

- Caution should be exercised when corticosteroids are to be used in the presence of recurrent, chronic, or acute infection.

Inflammation

When assaulted by physical, chemical, infective, or other assailants, the body reacts through the process of inflammation. Inflammation, characterized by the 4 cardinal signs of redness, heat, swelling, and pain, is the body's way of mobilizing its forces and defenses against the assault. The cardinal signs result as blood vessels dilate and more blood is pumped to the injured area. These blood vessels are leaky and allow specific cells and biochemicals to reach the site of injury. Tissue temperature increases to speed up cellular processes and begin repair.

Inflammation can be both a help and a hindrance. Though beneficial in fighting infection, its effects may be unwanted, as in the case of allergic reactions and specific autoimmune diseases.

The process of inflammation is the result of many different biochemical actions and interactions throughout the body. Many substances are produced or activated as a result of insult, including antibodies, specific white blood cells, proteins, and prostaglandins. Certain anti-inflammatory medications, like corticosteroids and nonsteroidal anti-inflammatory drugs (NSAIDs) work by interrupting these production and activation processes. Figure 7-1 demonstrates a specific example.

When signaled by injury to the body, certain biochemicals, called phospholipids, are converted into arachidonic acid. Arachidonic acid is then transformed by means of several separate pathways into other substances, one of which is prostaglandin. The prostaglandins and other substances are responsible for certain segments of the inflammatory process. Drugs such as corticosteroids and NSAIDs act at different levels of this process to prevent the formation of these biochemicals and their subsequent inflammatory effects.

Prostaglandins are regulatory chemicals of the inflammatory response. Their actions are dependent on the type of prostaglandin and the specific tissue on which it acts. In addition to pain and fever, prostaglandins play a role in the production of new blood vessels, clotting, gastric secretions, dilation and constriction of blood vessels, and uterine contractions, to name a few. In the eye, prostaglandins affect pain sensation, redness, and swelling. They may cause pupillary miosis during surgery and alter IOP.

As shown in Figure 7-1, corticosteroids block the production of arachidonic acid and prevent the formation of many different biochemicals, including prostaglandins. Acting more specifically, NSAIDs block only the production of the prostaglandins; other pathways are spared. In this manner, the corticosteroids and the NSAIDs act to decrease the pain, redness, and swelling associated with inflammation. Corticosteroids and NSAIDs do not, however, eliminate the stimulant causing the inflammation.

Corticosteroid Action

Corticosteroids are the workhorses of ophthalmic care when it comes to decreasing ocular inflammation. Whether the cause is mechanical, infective, chemical, or other, the actions of these therapeutics are the same.

Corticosteroids are related to and mimic substances produced by our own bodies. These substances have many action and control functions, only one of which is reduction of inflammation. As shown in Figure 7-1, corticosteroids affect the production of proteins, leukotrienes, and prostaglandins—all of which create various parts of the inflammatory response. In this manner, these drugs decrease dilation and permeability of blood vessels, thereby reducing the redness and swelling. They also decrease white blood cell proliferation, mast cell degranulation, and histamine release.

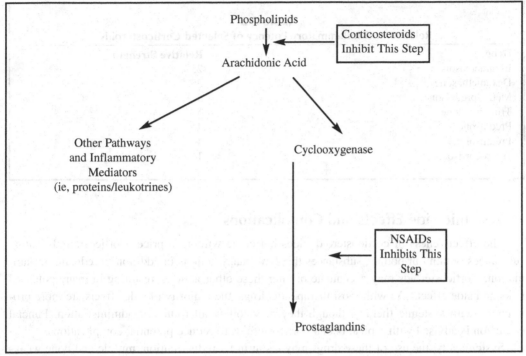

Figure 7-1. Interruption of the inflammatory process by corticosteroids and nonsteroidal anti-inflammatory drugs.

Table 7-1
Selected Uses for Corticosteroids in Ophthalmic Practice
Chemical Burns
Allergic Conjunctivitis
Immune Graft Reaction
Stromal Herpes Simplex Keratitis
Sterile Corneal Infiltration
Interstitial Keratitis
Uveitis
Scleritis/Episcleritis
Retinitis
Optic Neuritis
Temporal Arteritis
Orbital Pseudotumor
Graves' Ophthalmopathy

Due to their nonspecific action and overall effectiveness, corticosteroids are the most commonly used agents for reduction of ocular inflammation (Tables 7-1 and 7-2). They are also used in many other areas of medicine for a variety of systemic conditions.

Table 7-2
Relative Anti-Inflammatory Potency of Selected Corticosteroids

Drug	Relative Strength
Betamethasone	25
Dexamethasone	25
Methylprednisone	5
Triamcinolone	5
Prednisone	4
Prednisolone	4
Hydrocortisone	1

Systemic Side Effects and Complications

The effectiveness of corticosteroids does not come without a price. Corticosteroids mimic substances within our bodies, substances that have many actions in addition to reducing inflammation. Corticosteroids may accentuate or alter these other actions, resulting in many potential risks and side effects. As with most therapeutic drugs, the majority of side effects are more pronounced with systemic therapy, though they may follow all routes of administration. Punctal occlusion is advised with topical ocular corticosteroids to reduce potential complications.

Systemically, the use of these drugs may result in fat redistribution, muscle and bone weakness, fluid and electrolyte imbalances, growth retardation, stomach ulcers, and various psychoses. In addition, patients undergoing corticosteroid therapy become much more susceptible to a new or relapsing infection. This is especially true of herpetic infections. The reason is simply that the body's immune response is decreased during therapy. As a result, the body cannot mount a substantial defense against its attackers, and infections become more likely. Wound healing may also be delayed. Therefore, corticosteroids must be used cautiously in patients with active infection, a history of recurrent infection, or a decreased immune system.

Another major concern with the use of corticosteroids is adrenocortical insufficiency. The adrenal gland is an endocrine (hormone-producing) gland located on top of each kidney. The adrenal cortex produces corticosteroidlike chemicals. In adrenocortical insufficiency, there is a decrease or shutdown in the body's natural production of similar substances. Due to physiologic biofeedback, when corticosteroid therapy is used, the body senses the additional drug in the system. The body then decreases natural production in order to bring levels back into balance. When natural production is diminished over time, there may be atrophy (tissue death) of the adrenal cortex. If atrophy occurs, the body can no longer make the normal quantity of chemical itself, causing problems when the therapeutic dose is discontinued.

Adrenocortical insufficiency is usually temporary but can be permanent and is directly related to high doses and lengthy therapy. Adrenal suppression may be so severe that physiologic production cannot begin quickly enough when extended therapy is discontinued. Once withdrawal of the exogenous source has occurred, the required levels for normal body functions cannot be maintained. This can be a very dangerous situation. First, with inadequate levels of corticosteroids (physiologic or therapeutic), inflammation cannot be suppressed, and a rebound of the condition can occur. New organisms may also take advantage of the body's weakened state, and secondary problems can arise. Lastly, "steroid withdrawal" may cause symptoms of lethargy, weight loss, headache, fever, muscle soreness, nausea, and vomiting.

Because of the risks of stopping treatment prematurely, systemically administered cortico-steroids should not be discontinued abruptly if the length of therapy exceeds 5 to 7 days. Instead, therapy should be tapered by slowly reducing the dosage and frequency of administration. This allows physiologic levels to recover, thereby avoiding unwanted complications. The rate of withdrawal must correspond to the length and degree of therapy; the longer the course of treatment, the slower the withdrawal of the medication.

Suppression of adrenocortical function can occur but is rare with use of topical drops, and it is even less common with ointments and creams. Suppression is not expected after short-term topical therapy.

Ocular Side Effects and Complications

There are several potentially severe ocular side effects that can result from corticosteroid use. The first of these effects is the potential for development of posterior subcapsular cataracts. The nonreversible growth of these cataracts is directly related to the dosage and duration of treatment. Most cases are linked to prolonged treatment of 6 months or more with the more potent agents. Posterior subcapsular cataracts, because of their central location, can be visually debilitating and require surgical removal.

Secondly, topical corticosteroid therapy can cause an increase in IOP. Occurring in up to 8% 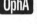 of individuals, elevated IOP is usually seen 3 to 6 weeks after initiation of treatment. Pressure ele-vation is seen more often with the use of more potent agents, such as dexamethasone, and more so in patients with preexisting glaucoma. Normally seen only after topical administration, it can arise from systemic use as well.

The increase in IOP is most likely the result of decreased aqueous outflow from the eye. It is not uncommon for sensitive individuals (called "steroid responders") to have pressure rises greater than 10 mm Hg. Any increase in IOP is generally reversible, returning to normal limits 1 to 3 weeks after discontinuation. However, if the IOP remains elevated for a length of time, so-called "steroid glaucoma" can occur with corresponding optic nerve damage and visual field loss. Patients on corticosteroid therapy must have their IOPs monitored on a regular basis to watch for these unwanted effects.

What the Patient Needs to Know

- Many adverse reactions are possible with corticosteroids. Any unusual changes should be reported to your physician.

- After using drops containing corticosteroids, close your eye and gently press your index finger against the corner of your eye (next to your nose). This helps keep the medicine on your eye and out of your system, decreasing the chances for side effects.

- Corticosteroid drops and ointments can cause glaucoma and cataracts. Faithful-ly keep every appointment with your eyecare practitioner, who can spot the early signs of these problems.

- The risk of cataracts and glaucoma from corticosteroid drops is minimal for the short period of use generally needed for most conditions.

- Never start steroid treatment without consulting a doctor.

- Never discontinue steroid therapy on your own. The medication needs to be tapered by the physician. Failure to do so can result in serious health risks.

Corticosteroid use can also lead to an increase in corneal thickness, mydriasis, and ptosis. As with systemic use, topical corticosteroid therapy should not be used alone in cases of acute infection. The anti-inflammatory properties will reduce associated symptoms, giving the appearance (to both doctor and patient) that the condition is resolving. In actuality, the drug is masking and aiding the progress of the underlying disease. In particular, corticosteroids should be used with caution when treating patients with a history of herpes simplex keratitis. These drugs can induce recurrences or exacerbate an existing episode.

Lastly, some commercial preparations contain sulfites. Certain patients have a known sensitivity to these compounds. Therefore, care must be exercised when choosing the therapeutic.

Administration

For ocular treatment, administration may be topical, injected (either directly or with close proximity to the desired site of action), intravenous, or oral.

Topical Corticosteroids

Topical administration is commonly the route of choice for ocular disorders. Most ocular inflammation manifests itself in the anterior segment of the eye: the conjunctiva, cornea, anterior chamber, and anterior uveal tract. In addition, topical administration decreases potential risks and side effects associated with these drugs.

In topical form, corticosteroids are the mainstay of therapy for inflammation involving the anterior segment of the eye. In addition to use after cataract or refractive surgery, there are many other uses for these agents. Topical corticosteroids work best in cases of acute inflammation and less well for chronic diseases. They have little, if any, effect on degenerative diseases.

Topical ophthalmic corticosteroids are available for administration as suspensions, solutions, and ointments. In some types, suspensions are more effective than solutions. Ointments are the least effective. Though they increase contact time with the ocular surface, ointments seem to bind the drug, decreasing availability for its intended use.

Each steroid base, such as prednisolone or dexamethasone, may be available in more than 1 form; for example, dexamethasone is available as dexamethasone alcohol or dexamethasone sodium phosphate. The alcohol or phosphate form is known as its derivative. The derivative of the corticosteroid has an important role in both its overall effect and its vehicle. In therapeutic mixtures, acetate and alcohol formulations will form suspensions, while phosphate preparations will remain true solutions. Furthermore, given the same corticosteroid base, acetate preparations have more anti-inflammatory activity than alcohols; phosphate preparations are yet less effective. The choice of which steroid to use is made weighing the relative cost, convenience, safety, and effectiveness of the available corticosteroids (Table 7-3) against the patient's condition and need for treatment.

Frequency of application may be as often as every hour to once a day, depending on the type, location, severity, and course of the inflammatory condition. Therapy should be started quickly and aggressively enough to suppress the inflammation. Once the inflammation is quelled, tapering should begin.

Normally, it is not necessary to taper after topical ocular therapy unless the duration of treatment exceeds 2 or 3 weeks or the inflammation was severe. In these cases, the physician may prefer to use a short tapering period: 4 times per day for 4 days, 3 times per day for 3 days, and so

Table 7-3
Effectiveness in Reduction of Corneal Inflammation of Selected Topical Corticosteroids

Drug	Decrease Through Intact Epithelium
Prednisolone Acetate 1%	51%
Dexamethasone 0.1%	40%
Fluorometholone 0.1%	31%
Prednisolone phosphate 1%	28%
Dexamethasone phosphate 0.1%	18%

on until discontinuing the medication entirely. If used long-term or with recurrent disease, slower tapering is necessary (decreasing by only 1 drop per week or slower). Patients must always be cautioned of the dangers of discontinuing corticosteroids on their own accord.

Injections and Intravenous Injections

Periocular injection is used in cases where inflammation is not responding to drops alone and additional help is needed. The drug is usually injected just below the conjunctiva or in the space below Tenon's capsule. Here, more absorption will occur, and more drug will be made available to the desired site. Periocular injection is additive to topical therapy but lacks the efficacy, convenience, and safety to be considered a first-line treatment.

It is sometimes advantageous to inject the drug directly into a lesion. This is particularly true when treating chalazia (inflammatory lesions of the eyelids). Betamethasone (Celestone®) and triancinolone (Aristocert®, Kenacort®) are primarily the agents of choice for this route of administration.

Management of certain ocular conditions sometimes calls for intravenous corticosteroids. Recently, the intravenous use of methylprednisone, in combination with oral corticosteroids, has become accepted treatment in severe cases of optic neuritis.

Oral Administration

Oral administration, usually prednisone, is used infrequently in ophthalmic care. Its major role is in the treatment of ocular inflammation resulting from systemic diseases—such as Grave's disease, myasthenia gravis, and temporal arteritis—and collagen vascular diseases, such as rheumatoid arthritis. In most cases, both topical and periocular administration are safer and more effective options. Occasionally, however, in the treatment of severe anterior segment inflammation or posterior segment involvement, oral administration (alone or in conjunction with other routes) is warranted.

Types of Corticosteroids   OphT

The most commonly used corticosteroids for topical ocular use are prednisolone, fluorometholone, dexamethasone, rimexolone, and medrysone.

Prednisolone

Prednisolone acetate 1% (Pred Forte®, Econopred Plus®) is considered the standard by which all other topical ocular corticosteroids are compared. This suspension crosses the cornea more easily and has the greatest efficacy when compared to all other available ophthalmic agents. As such, it is more likely to elevate IOP and have greater side effects than its weaker counterparts. For this reason, most practitioners either use weaker prednisolone 0.12% or 0.125% suspensions (PredMild®, Econopred®) or totally shun this agent when treating mild cases of inflammation. Prednisolone sodium phosphate solutions are also available. They are marketed as solutions in 1% (Ak-Pred®, Inflamase Forte®) and 0.125% concentrations (Ak-Pred®, Inflamase®). Prednisolone is not available as an ophthalmic ointment.

Fluorometholone

Fluorometholone is available as both a suspension and an ointment. Marketed in a 0.1% concentration as both a suspension (Fluor-op®, FML®) and ointment (FML S.O.P.®), and as a 0.25% suspension (FML Forte®), this relatively weaker corticosteroid is used primarily in the treatment of mild to moderate forms of chronic inflammation (usually allergic conjunctivitis). It lacks the efficacy to be used satisfactorily in cases of uveitis. The benefit derived from these medications is the decreased risk of unwanted complications, such as IOP rise.

A more recent introduction to the therapeutic arsenal has been the addition of fluorometholone acetate suspension in a 0.1% concentration (Flarex®, Eflone®). Due to its acetate formulation, movement across the cornea is much improved, increasing its effectiveness. Studies indicate that it approaches the efficacy of prednisolone acetate but is less likely to cause IOP rise. It may be the treatment of choice in those patients with a history of pressure rise due to corticosteroid therapy or previously diagnosed glaucoma. Of course, all of the corticosteroids are capable of increasing IOP, and patients on long-term therapy (even those on "safer" medications) must have their IOPs measured regularly.

Dexamethasone

Dexamethasone is a potent corticosteroid available as a 0.1% sodium phosphate solution (Ak-Dex®, Baldex®, Decadron®, Dexotic®) and a 0.1% suspension (Maxidex®). It is also available as a 0.05% ophthalmic ointment (AK-Dex®, Baldex®, Decadron®, Maxidex®). Dexamethasone is very effective in reducing ocular inflammation, but it has the propensity to increase IOP more than any other topical ophthalmic corticosteroid. For this reason, it is usually limited to short course therapy or as an alternative when other corticosteroids are not available. When applied at bedtime, dexamethasone ointment is very useful for nighttime coverage in cases of uveitis. Combined with an antibiotic, it is also popular for the reduction of inflammation after cataract or refractive surgery.

Rimexolone

Rimexolone 1% ophthalmic suspension (Vexol®) is indicated for use postoperatively and in cases of anterior segment inflammation. The main advantage of this drug is that it has more of a site-specific action than other corticosteroids. In other words, the majority of its action occurs at the site where it is applied and less so elsewhere. Thus, while having efficacy similar to prednisolone acetate 1%, it has less tendency to increase the IOP. Due to its limited systemic absorption, it is also less likely to cause adverse adrenocortical effects. For these reasons, rimexolone is a valuable addition to the armamentarium against ocular inflammation.

Medrysone

Marketed as a 1% suspension (HMS®), this corticosteroid has the least anti-inflammatory effect of all available therapeutics in this class. It is useful only in mild inflammatory conditions and not in cases of uveitis. Because of its relatively weak strength, it has very little systemic effect and elevates IOP minimally or not at all. Though some practitioners feel it has a niche in treating allergic conjunctivitis, these authors feel that newer nonsteroidal anti-inflammatory agents work better to reduce inflammation with less potential for adverse effects; all in all, it is a very limited drug with very limited use.

Loteprednol

Loteprednol etabonate ophthalmic suspension (Alrex®, Lotemax®) 0.2% and 0.5% is a less potent steroid indicated for temporary relief of the signs and symptoms of seasonal allergic conjunctivitis. Because it is a suspension, it needs to be shaken vigorously before use. It is less effective in cases requiring more potent steroid activity, such as deep-seated inflammatory diseases.

Bibliography

Barlett JD, Jaanus SD. *Clinical Ocular Pharmacology*. 2nd ed. Stoneham, Mass: Buttersworth; 1980.

Bohigian, GM. *Handbook of External Diseases of the Eye*. 2nd ed. St. Louis, Mo: DAC Medical Publishing Assoc; 1980.

Ellis PP. *Ocular Therapeutic and Pharmacology*. 6th ed. St. Louis, Mo: CV Mosby; 1981.

Lewis LL, Fingeret M. *Primary Care of the Glaucomas*. East Norwalk, Conn: Appleton and Lange; 1993.

Kumar V, Cotran RS, Robbins SL. *Basic Pathology*. 5th ed. Philadelphia, Pa: WB Saunders; 1992.

Marielo EN. *Human Anatomy & Physiology*. Redwood City, Calif: Benjamin/Cummings Publishing; 1980.

Melton R, Thomas R. *4th Annual Guide to Therapeutic Drugs*. Norwalk, Conn: Optometric Management; May 1995.

Moses RA, Hart WN Jr. *Adler's Physiology of the Eye: Clinical Application*. 8th ed. St. Louis, Mo: CV Mosby; 1987.

Onofrey BE. *Clinical Optometric Pharmacology & Therapeutics*. Philadelphia, Pa: JB Lippincott; 1992.

Ophthalmic Drug Facts. St. Louis, Mo: JB Lippincott; 1990.

PDR for Ophthalmology. 23rd ed. Montauk, NJ: Medical Economics Books; 1995.

Silverman HM, ed. *The Pill Book*. 6th ed. New York, NY: Bantam Books; 1994.

Chapter 8

Nonsteroidal Anti-Inflammatory Drugs (NSAIDs)

- NSAIDs are generally less potent anti-inflammatory agents than corticosteroids and have fewer adverse effects. This makes them a better alternative where chronic use is indicated.

- Oral NSAIDs are readily available and are effective for reducing pain, fever, and inflammation arising from a variety of causes.

- Acetaminophen, though classified with the NSAIDs and used in reducing pain and fever, has no anti-inflammatory effect.

- Topical NSAIDs work very well in reducing the pain associated with corneal injuries such as an abrasion or keratorefractive surgery.

Introduction

Turn on the television, and you will recognize athletes and celebrities proclaiming the benefits of these "wonder drugs." Known as nonsteroidal anti-inflammatory drugs (NSAIDs), the brand names are known instantly: Bayer®, Bufferin®, Tylenol®, Advil®, and the list goes on.

Derivatives of aspirin, the NSAIDs are probably the most commonly administered drugs. In tablet form, they can be purchased OTC or by prescription for use in many conditions. Now, topical NSAIDs are quickly gaining acceptance and popularity for their effectiveness in ophthalmic practice.

Systemically, NSAIDs decrease fever, pain, and inflammation. In the last chapter, we discussed the process of inflammation. (You may want to glance at Figure 7-1 to review.) Both corticosteroids and NSAIDs reduce inflammation. Whereas corticosteroids act in a general manner to decrease production of several biochemicals, NSAIDs *specifically* reduce the production of the prostaglandins. This is accomplished by inhibiting a specific substance called cyclooxygenase, which is needed to make prostaglandins. The action of the NSAIDs is, thus, much more specific; other routes are not affected and are available to respond as needed.

Fever is one result of inflammation. The increasing temperature speeds up the body's metabolism, enabling the body to fight disease and repair injury. NSAIDs act to lower elevated body temperature. This is known as an antipyretic effect, which corticosteroids do not have. NSAIDs do not lower body temperature unless there is a fever.

The role of NSAIDs in reducing pain is not yet completely understood. However, it has been shown that the pain-reducing effect, called analgesia, is not linked to the anti-inflammatory effect; that is, the dose needed to decrease pain is less than that needed to decrease inflammation. Lastly, NSAIDs also inhibit the blood's ability to clot and prolong bleeding time. This effect is best known by the well-publicized role of aspirin in reducing the chance of stroke and second heart attack.

Compared with the corticosteroids, NSAIDs are less potent. In turn, they have fewer side effects and fewer adverse reactions. Due to their specific mode of action, many concerns of corticosteroid therapy, such as adrenocortical insufficiency, are not present with NSAIDs. The most common adverse effects are gastrointestinal in nature: stomach upset, vomiting, and ulceration. NSAIDs may also induce kidney dysfunction and promote asthma. These therapeutics must be used with care in patients susceptible to these complications and those with reduced clotting ability.

What the Patient Needs to Know

- Use oral NSAIDs with caution if you have stomach or digestive problems or are susceptible to prolonged bleeding.

- Acetaminophen has no anti-inflammatory effect but is good for pain and fever.

- Aspirin should not be used in teens or adolescents with flulike symptoms. (Acetaminophen is a good alternative.)

- NSAID eye drops sting when you put them in.

Table 8-1
Selected Oral NSAIDs

Drug	Brand Name
aspirin	Bayer, Bufferin
acetaminophen (non-NSAID)	Tylenol
diclofenac	Voltaren
diflusinal	Dolobid
flurbiprofen	Ansaid
ibuprofen	Advil, Motrin,
Nuprin	
indomethacin	Indocin
ketoprofen	Orudis
ketorolac	Toradol
naproxen	Anaprox,
Naprosyn, Aleve	
piroxicam	Feldene

Nonprescription NSAIDs are effective in reducing the normal joint and muscle pain after strenuous activity and aid in the relief of flulike symptoms and headache. In stronger doses, NSAIDs are used to treat chronic inflammation associated with conditions like rheumatoid arthritis and lupus.

Due to their anti-inflammatory properties, both oral and topical NSAIDs should never be used alone in the presence of an acute infection because they can dangerously mask and aid the infection's progress.

Oral Administration

The indications for orally administered NSAIDs in ophthalmic practice are few. These agents are mostly used for relief of mild to moderate pain after ocular surgery. They are generally not effective for significantly reducing the pain associated with corneal injury. NSAIDs are available by prescription in combination with narcotics for additional pain relief. Orally and topically, NSAIDs may be useful for treating idiopathic central serous chorioretinopathy (ICSC) and cystoid macular edema (CME); these are inflammatory conditions resulting in fluid accumulation in the retina.

Though all NSAIDs are pharmacologically similar and have like actions, they possess slightly different characteristics, which set them apart from one another. Some of the more commonly prescribed oral NSAIDs for ophthalmic use are aspirin, ibuprofen, ketorolac, acetaminophen, and indomethacin (Table 8-1). Having these and many other agents at our disposal, the proper selection of a drug is based on their slightly varied characteristics, physician preference and familiarity, the condition being treated, and the desired effect.

Aspirin

Aspirin is the oldest and most well known of all the NSAIDs, and it is considered the standard measure for all drugs in this class. It possesses the anti-inflammatory, antipyretic, and analgesic properties common to these drugs. Aspirin does have a high incidence of adverse effects, most commonly gastrointestinal disorders. However, its track record and effectiveness maintains its popularity. Aspirin should not be administered to adolescents or teens with flulike symptoms due to its association with Reye's syndrome, a potentially fatal condition.

Acetaminophen

Acetaminophen (Tylenol®) is technically not a true NSAID because it possesses no anti-inflammatory activity. It is a weak prostaglandin inhibitor but has considerable ability to reduce pain and fever; thus, it has been grouped with the NSAIDs. Acetaminophen is a very safe drug when taken in recommended doses, having very few side effects or adverse reactions. It is a very good alternative to aspirin and other NSAIDs in reducing pain and fever, when those drugs are contraindicated.

Ibuprofen

Ibuprofen is another commonly administered drug. It has similar anti-inflammatory and adverse effects as aspirin. Like all NSAIDs, it can prolong bleeding time and should be used cautiously in susceptible patients. The tendency to reduce clotting is, however, less than that exhibited by aspirin.

Indomethacin

Indomethacin deserves special mention because of its history in treating various ocular conditions. It has proven effective in reducing inflammation associated with some cases of CME, ICSC, uveitis, and optic neuritis. Its usefulness in the treatment of these conditions has not been fully established, and it is not universally accepted. In other conditions, there are better options available. Indomethacin is a very potent inhibitor of prostaglandins and is extremely effective. Added to its effectiveness is a high rate of adverse reactions—more than any other of its counterparts. Nausea, gastrointestinal complications, and central nervous system disorders (such as dizziness, headache, depression, and fatigue) are not uncommon. It has been estimated that up to 50% of patients on indomethacin therapy experience adverse reactions; 20% must discontinue use as a result.

Ketorolac

Finally, ketorolac has an increased analgesic effect that some clinicians say rivals the acetaminophen/narcotic combination. The increased analgesic effect of ketolorac may be potent enough to significantly diminish the pain associated with corneal injuries, abrasions, and various keratopathies. However, it should not be used for more than 15 days due to the severity of possible side effects.

Ocular Administration

Topical administration of NSAIDs has been approved for 3 clinical implications in ophthalmic care: the reduction of postoperative inflammation, the relief of itching in allergic conjunctivitis, and the prevention of pupillary miosis during surgery. Topical NSAIDs have also been proven effective in reducing the pain of corneal surgery and may have a role in other ocular inflammatory conditions. Though each has specific approved uses, all have similar activities. No doubt, as we learn and understand more about these relatively new ophthalmic drugs, their indications will grow.

Topical use of NSAIDs is relatively free of adverse effects, the exception being stinging on instillation. Unlike corticosteroids, there does not appear to be significant elevation in IOP, even following prolonged treatment. Again, caution must be exercised in patients where prolonged bleeding could lead to complications, such as the formation of hyphema.

Flurbiprofen and Suprofen

Srg

Flurbiprofen sodium 0.03% (Ocufen®) and suprofen (Profenal®) are similar topical NSAIDs. The main indication for each is the inhibition of miosis during intraocular surgery. As a result of trauma, surgery in this case, prostaglandins are released within the eye, producing a miotic response. Ocufen and Profenal block prostaglandin release and prohibit the unwanted miosis. Though officially approved only for prevention of miosis, Ocufen has been used in cases of mild uveitis, postsurgical inflammation, and the treatment of CME with varied success.

Ocufen is administered as a single drop every 30 minutes for 2 hours before surgery. Administration of Profenal begins the day before surgery: 2 drops every 4 hours. On the day of surgery, 2 drops are placed in the eye 3, 2, and 1 hour(s) before the procedure.

Diclofenac

Diclofenac ophthalmic solution 0.1% (Voltaren®) has been approved for the treatment of postoperative inflammation after cataract surgery. No other topical NSAID is as effective at inhibiting prostaglandin synthesis. Voltaren also works well in the management of corneal pain. It is often used before patching a corneal abrasion or in conjunction with an antibiotic when patching is not necessary. Diclofenac is also becoming incorporated into the standard protocol after keratorefractive surgery (particularly photorefractive keratectomy). In this case, 1 or 2 drops are instilled into the eye before surgery and then 4 times daily until the cornea is re-epithelialized. After cataract surgery, standard application is 1 drop 4 times daily beginning 24 hours postoperatively and sustained over a period of 2 weeks. Transient burning is reported in up to 15% of patients treated.

Ketorolac

Ketorolac tromethamine 0.5% solution (Acular®) is the only topical NSAID approved for use in treating the itching associated with allergic conjunctivitis. Due to its safety when compared to the corticosteroids, it is becoming the first choice of many when treating mild or moderate itching. For this application, Acular is instilled 4 times daily. Though its efficacy beyond 1 week has not been studied, clinical experience has shown no decrease in effectiveness or increase in adverse reaction over a course of several weeks. Transient stinging is common, reported in up to 40% of patients.

Acular, like the other topical NSAIDs, is clinically effective in managing corneal pain. It is reported that Acular's ability to reduce pain and itch may stem from an ability to raise the sensory threshold. In other words, sensitivity to the painful stimulus is lessened to the point where it is no longer bothersome and the eye feels "normal." When used after corneal injury or surgery, Acular significantly reduces patient discomfort. Over time, this use as an analgesic may emerge as the major ophthalmic role of these agents.

Bibliography

Barlett JD, Jaanus SD. *Clinical Ocular Pharmacology*. 2nd ed. Stoneham, Mass: Butterworths; 1980.

Ellis PP. *Ocular Therapeutics and Pharmacology*. 6th ed. St. Louis, Mo: CV Mosby; 1981.

Kumar V, Cotran RS, Robbins SC. *Basic Pathology*. 5th ed. Philadelphia, Pa: WB Saunders; 1992.

Marielo EN. *Human Anatomy & Physiology*. Redwood City, Calif: Benjamin/Cummings Publishing; 1980.

Melton R, Thomas R. 4th Annual guide to therapeutic drugs. *Optometric Management*. May 1995.

Moses RA, Hart WH Jr. *Adler's Physiology of the Eye: Clinical Application*. 5th ed. St. Louis, Mo: CV Mosby; 1987.

Onofrey BE. *Clinical Optometric Pharmacology and Therapeutics*. Philadelphia, Pa: JB Lippincott; 1992.

Ophthalmic Drug Facts. St. Louis, Mo: JB Lippincott; 1990.

PDR for Ophthalmology. 23rd ed. Montauk, NJ: Medical Economics; 1995.

Shenan PW. A practical guide to allergy medications. *Review of Ophthalmology*. 1996; 3(3):112-117.

Silverman HM, ed. *The Pill Book*. 6th ed. New York, NY: Bantam Books; 1994.

Chapter 9

Anesthetics

Introduction

Sensation to the upper eyelids and brows is provided by the first division of the trigeminal nerve (cranial nerve V). This nerve also provides sensation to the upper bulbar conjunctiva and superior cornea. The second division of the trigeminal nerve supplies sensory input to the lower eyelids and a small portion of the inferior cornea and lower bulbar conjunctiva.

An anesthetic is a medication that eliminates sensation. General anesthetics are usually administered by IV or inhalation for the purpose of inducing sleep and eliminating pain. In ophthalmology, general anesthesia is rarely used but does have a place in physically or emotionally traumatic surgeries. A discussion of general anesthesia is beyond the scope of this book. Procedures performed on the eye and its adnexa are best approached with various forms of regional (or local) anesthetics. Anesthesia can be obtained by blocking the sensory nerves that serve the eye and the skin of the eyelids and surrounding tissues. This type of anesthesia is appropriately called a "block." Local anesthesia can also be achieved on a short-term basis by injecting the tissue directly, without blocking the supplying nerve. In addition, because the surface of the eye is exposed, it can be anesthetized directly with the use of eye drops (topical anesthesia) (Table 9-1). Besides providing impairment of sensory information to block the perception of pain, surgeons often wish to immobilize the muscles of the eyelid and extraocular muscles. Thus, a secondary function of anesthetic is impairment of movement. This can be accomplished by a retrobulbar block: injecting anesthesia into the muscle cone and allowing dissipation of the anesthetic to the optic nerve and the second, third, fourth, and fifth cranial nerves.

Mechanism of Action

All anesthetics work by blocking the transmission of neural impulses from the naked nerve endings in the eyelid skin, conjunctiva, or cornea to the nerve cell body and back to the brain. Chemically, this occurs by blocking sodium channels and preventing depolarization of the nerve, therefore, preventing the physiologic conduction of the impulse.

Depending on the formulation of the anesthetic, the onset of the action and its duration can be controlled. First, the more rapidly that the anesthetic is metabolized, the shorter acting it is; the longer acting anesthetics can last for several hours. The duration of action of the local anesthetic is related to the physiologic effect of that anesthetic, as well. In small concentrations, most local anesthetics cause constriction of blood vessels, which slows the breakdown of the anesthetic. At higher concentrations and volumes, a reverse dilation of vessels occurs, which facilitates more rapid breakdown of the drug.

Systemic Toxicity

All anesthetics have a potential to become toxic in higher doses. Individuals may experience lightheadedness, ringing in their ears, or blurred vision. At even higher doses, respiratory arrest can occur, as well as convulsions, coma, and death. Preventing the absorption of the drug by the vessels will minimize the concentration of the drug in the systemic circulation, reducing the likelihood of toxicity. In locally injected anesthetics, this is accomplished by using a vasoconstrictor, such as epinephrine. When topical anesthetic is used, punctal occlusion can reduce the amount of drug that is absorbed into the system.

Table 9-1
Selected Anesthetics

Topical
Proparacaine HCL	5% (Alcane®, Ocucaine®, AKTaine®)
Tetracaine HCL	0.5% (Cetacaine®)

Injectable
Bupivacaine	0.25% to 0.75% (Marcaine®)
Etidocaine	1%
Lidocaine	1% to 2% (Xylocaine®, Dalcaine®)
Mepivacaine	1% to 2% (Carbocaine®)
Prilocaine	1% to 2%
Procaine	1% to 4% (Novocain®)

Anesthetic Adjuncts

Anesthesia usually produces blockage of the sensation of pain. However, the ability to move and sensation of pressure may still exist. Accordingly, many surgeons choose to use supplemental sedation, such as anxiolytics or hypnotics, to increase the effectiveness of the local anesthetic. These may be administered orally before surgery or intravenously at the time of surgery.

Anesthetic Agents

Local anesthetics can be divided into 2 chemical groups: the amides and the esters. Amide anesthetics, because of their chemical structure, can penetrate fat-soluble tissues as well as water-soluble tissues, making them ideal for application to the surface of the eye. Common examples of the amide anesthetics include lidocaine, xylocaine, ultracaine, etidocane, duranest, mepivacaine, carbocaine, policaine, bupivacaine, marcaine, sensorcaine, and ropivacaine.
The ester group of anesthetics is commonly associated with increased allergies and, therefore, is generally used only in topical form, as opposed to injection. Common examples of ester anesthetics include cocaine, procaine, novocaine, tetracaine, pontocaine, proparacaine, ophthaine, ophthetic, alcaine, benoxinate, and dorsacaine. Cocaine was used as a topical anesthetic for eye surgery dating back to the 1800s. Because of its potential for toxicity, both in the eye and systematically, cocaine is not commonly used today.

Administration of Anesthetic Agents

Injection

Typically, one of the amide anesthetics is combined with a longer-acting ester anesthetic to provide long-acting motor and sensory anesthesia. These mixtures can be injected directly into the muscle cone of the orbit, blocking the motor and sensory nerves of the eye. Injection of anesthetic can also be given directly into the orbicularis muscles of the eyelid (Van Lint block), into the

---

What the Patient Needs to Know

- You are being given a local anesthetic to numb the area the doctor will be working on.

- The numbness will last ____.

- If, during or after the injection, you feel pain, notify the physician.

- When the anesthetic wears off, you may feel sore where the injection was given or a tingling sensation in the tissues.

- Although anesthetics minimize pain, they do not eliminate sensation. Expect feelings of touch and pressure.

---

seventh nerve as it crosses the maxillary bone, for a nerve block (O'Brien block), or directly into the stylomastoid foramen, for complete motor block of the facial muscles on that side (Atkinson block).

 Because injection requires blind passage of a needle into soft tissue, there are associated risks. These commonly include the rupture of vessels causing a retrobulbar hemorrhage, damage to extraocular muscles or nerves, perforation of the globe itself, or inadvertent injection of the anesthetic into the aural space, causing suppression of respiration or heart rate. Allergic reactions to the anesthetic itself can also occur, including anaphylactic shock. Therefore, access to resuscitative equipment is always required when injection of anesthesia is planned. Injection of anesthetics into the orbital area is never to be taken lightly and should be performed only by a physician, anesthesiologist, or specially trained individual who recognizes these potential hazards. The administration of an anesthetic should always be part of any informed consent discussion for surgery. Figure 9-1 demonstrates the administration of a retrobulbar anesthetic.

Lidocaine is the most widely used injectable. For longer duration, bupivacaine is used.

 ## Topical Anesthesia

Topical anesthetics are used in ophthalmology for a variety of other purposes. Any test requiring contact with the cornea is made more comfortable if topical anesthetic is used first. Indeed, some of these tests would be nearly impossible for the patient to endure if the cornea was not numbed first. These tests include tonometry, pachymetry, ultrasound, and specular microscopy (cell count). Certain tear function tests are performed with topical anesthesia, as well. It is important to note that certain tests, such as corneal sensation, must be performed without topical anesthesia. Another use of numbing drops is to reduce the stinging sensation of dilating drops.

In addition to numbing the cornea and conjunctiva for testing, topical anesthetic is required in procedures such as removal of a foreign body or scraping a corneal lesion. In these cases, a drop may be applied directly to the area once a minute for 5 minutes for maximum anesthesia. Radial keratotomy and other refractive surgical procedures are commonly performed using only topical anesthesia. It is also becoming popular to perform cataract surgery with topical anesthetic. Figure 9-2 demonstrates the administration of a topical anesthetic eye drop.

Tetracaine is the most popular topical anesthetic and is available for single use in dropper bottles or ampules. Tetracaine is unpreserved. Proparacaine and benoxinate contain preservatives and are effective in anesthetizing the corneal nerve endings through topical application. These formulations are highly osmotic and, therefore, sting and burn when applied. Sometimes,

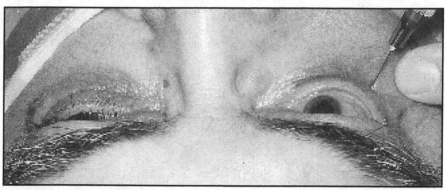

Figure 9-1. Delivery of retrobulbar anesthetic.

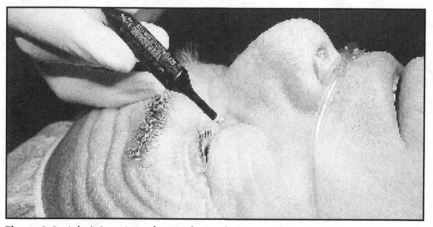

Figure 9-2. Administration of topical anesthetic eye drops.

diluting the topical anesthetic with balanced salt solution can decrease the discomfort when the first drop is instilled. Once the drop has made contact with the eye, however, anesthesia is obtained, and subsequent drops generally are not uncomfortable.

Topical anesthetic drops are never prescribed for a patient to use at home. Frequent use interferes with the healing process and can cause corneal melting. In-office use for testing and procedures is not usually risky, but unmonitored use for control of pain is contraindicated. In addition, patients should be warned not to rub their eyes after instillation of topical anesthetics. Because the cornea now lacks sensation, the patient could conceivably rub hard enough to cause a corneal abrasion.

What the Patient Needs to Know

- This drop will numb your eye for _____ minutes while the test or procedure is being performed.

- Please do not rub your eye while it is numb, because you might scratch it accidentally.

- The first drop may sting, but you should not feel other drops after that.

- These drops cannot be prescribed for home use because they interfere with healing when used on a regular basis.

Bibliography

Fine IH, Fichman RA, Grabow HB. *Clear Corneal Cataract Surgery and Topical Anesthesia*. Thorofare, NJ: Slack Incorporated; 1993.

Gills JP, Hustead RF, Sanders DR. *Ophthalmic Anesthesia*. Thorofare, NJ: Slack Incorporated; 1993.

Anti-Infectives

- Most common ocular infections can be treated topically, although systemic treatment may be indicated for lid, orbital, and posterior segment involvement.

- A "shotgun" approach to treating ocular infection is not recommended. Therapy should be directed specifically at the causative organism. Cultures and drug sensitivities should be obtained when necessary.

- Anti-infectives must be used responsibly. Overuse can result in the development of resistant organisms. Highly potent agents, such as fluoroquinolones, should be reserved for more serious infections to avoid resistance and maintain effectiveness.

- Infections that do not resolve after an appropriate length of therapy may be the result of targeting the wrong organism, using an improper agent, or the development of resistance. Consider, also, a possible allergic or toxic response to the medication.

Infection

Infection occurs when the body's defenses are overcome and injured by a microorganism. Infections can be caused by bacteria, parasites, viruses, and fungi. Given the number of these microorganisms we are in contact with every day, the number of resulting infections is remarkably low. This is because the body has many barriers to infection. These barriers are both nonspecific and specific. Nonspecific defenses include physical barriers provided by skin, membranes, and secretions (such as mucous and stomach acid). These barriers are very effective. For example, there are only a handful of bacteria that are capable of causing corneal infection as long as the outer surface of the cornea—the epithelium—remains intact. Secondly, the body's immune system has defenses against a specific microorganism, should nonspecific measures fail to contain it. When a microorganism breeches these defenses, infection results. Infections can occur in any tissues, including those of the eye.

In some cases, physical barriers may not work. For example, if the eye becomes scratched and the epithelium is damaged, that person is more likely to develop infection. The same is true after surgery, where physical barriers are purposely broken.

Certain individuals are more susceptible to getting infections. Diabetics and individuals who are immunocompromised have a poorly functioning immune system and cannot use their specific defenses efficiently. This can be the result of another disease, such as the human immunodeficiency virus, the virus causing autoimmune deficiency syndrome (AIDS). Immunodeficiency can also be caused by medications, such as corticosteroids.

Whatever the reason, when an infection occurs, anti-infective therapy should be instituted. Therapy may include antibacterials, antivirals, antifungals, or antiparasitics. For these drugs to be effective, they must be able to eliminate the microorganism while causing as little damage as possible to the human host. The ability to target the microorganism rather than the host is known as selective toxicity. This is accomplished by designing drugs that work on characteristics particular to a certain microorganism. Bacteria, fungi, viruses, and parasites all have features that are unique unto themselves. By targeting those unique qualities, we can act on the infectious organism, while causing as little harm as possible to the other cells of the body.

Antibacterial Therapy

When the cause of an infection is presumed or proven to be bacterial, antibacterial drugs are used to stop it. Antibacterial drugs can be either bactericidal or bacteriostatic. A bactericidal drug directly kills the bacteria. In contrast, a bacteriostatic drug keeps the bacteria from multiplying, holding it in check until our own defenses can eliminate it. Bactericidal drugs are usually preferred over bacteriostatic ones. Antibacterial drugs can work in a variety of ways to accomplish their goal. They can disrupt the wall of the cell, alter cellular membranes or protein production, disrupt synthesis of vital components, or alter cellular DNA.

Not all bacteria are susceptible to every antibacterial drug. Some drugs may be bacteriocidal to some organisms and bacteriostatic to others; other bacteria may not be affected at all. The range of bacteria that a drug is effective in eliminating is known as that drug's spectrum of action. A drug that has a broad spectrum is effective against a wide range of bacteria. A drug with a narrow spectrum affects only a few species of bacteria.

Bacteria can be classified according to the structure of their cell walls. A common way to do this classification is to use the gram stain test. In this test, a slide is smeared with bacteria and flooded with gram stain. Based on the structure of the cell wall, the bacteria stains a certain color and is then classified as either gram positive or gram negative. Certain antibiotics affect mainly gram-positive organisms while others affect mainly gram-negative organisms. Some drugs affect both. However, a drug can be effective against most bacteria in a certain class and be ineffective against a few others in that same category. It is always wise to obtain a culture to determine which bacteria is causing the infection. Once this is known, an antibiotic effective against that organism is selected.

Certain bacteria are more common than others in ophthalmic practice. Examples of gram-positive organisms important in ocular infections include *Staphylococcus aureus*, *Staphylococcus epidermidis*, and *Streptococcus pneumoniae*. Examples of gram-negative bacteria are *Neisseria gonorrhea*, *Haemophilus influenzae*, and *Pseudomonas aeruginosa*. It should be noted here that the treatment of certain other infections involving acanthamoeba (a protozoan) and parasites (eg, *Toxoplasmosis gondii* and *Chlamydia trachomatis*) are often treated with antibacterial drugs. These infectious organisms may share common physiologic properties with bacteria; thus, antibacterial drugs are sometimes used in the management of nonbacterial infections.

A commonly occurring problem is that bacteria that were once susceptible to the actions of a certain drug can develop resistance to this agent over time. After exposure to a drug, bacteria can become resistant through mutation, selection, and adaptation. This resistance is becoming widespread, making some other drugs, once very effective, now of much less value. This is one reason the production of new pharmaceuticals is necessary.

Like other drugs, administration of antibiotics may be by way of injection (intravenous or local), orally, or topically depending on the location, duration, severity, and type of infection. Most ocular infections are superficial and involve the conjunctiva and cornea. Topical administration by drop or ointment is preferred—usually 1 drop 2 to 4 times a day but up to 1 drop every

What the Patient Needs to Know

- Always follow doctors' instructions when taking anti-infectives. Using drops more often than prescribed may cause a toxic reaction. If you use too little, the infection may be prolonged.

- Always finish the full course of anti-infective therapy. Discontinuing medication too soon may result in the infection coming back.

- Stomach upset is very common with oral antibiotic therapy. This does not mean you are allergic to the medication. Ask your doctor if "cultured" food like yogurt can be eaten to reduce this upset.

- Never use nonophthalmic OTC antibiotics in the eye. They are meant for skin, not eyes. Always use approved eye drops unless instructed by your physician.

- Tetracycline products may increase your sensitivity to the sun. Beware of sunburn.

- As a general rule, tetracyclines should not be taken with dairy products or antacids. This may reduce their effectiveness.

- Certain antibacterial drops sting briefly when you put them in. If they sting for a prolonged time, notify your physician.

- Vigamox® is naturally yellow colored; this does not mean that the drops have gone bad.

Table 10-1
Selected Combination Antibiotic Ointments (Brand Names)

Polymixin B/Neomycin/Bacitracin
Neotal
Neotracin
Triple Antibiotic
Ak-Spore
Neosporin

Polymixin/Bacitracin
Ak-Poly-Bac
Polysporin

Polymixin B/Neomycin
Statrol

Selected Combination Antibiotic Solutions (Brand Names)

Polymixin B/Neomycin
Statrol

Polymixin B/Neomycin/Gramicidin
Ak-Spore
Neosporin
Neotracin

Polymixin B/Trimethoprim
Polytrim

hour with more severe corneal involvement. Deeper infections of the lid, periorbital tissue, or lacrimal drainage system often require oral administration. Intraocular infections are rare but can occur after penetrating injury or surgery. This is an emergency situation. Patients are hospitalized and given topical, intravenous, periocular, and oral antibiotic therapy.

Combination Antibiotics

Combination antibiotics are popular and numerous in ophthalmic practice (Table 10-1). The advantage of these mixtures is that the combination of 2 or more drugs enhances the overall activity of the preparation. Two drugs with narrow and differing spectrums can be combined to form a combination with a broad overall spectrum. This may have advantages in prophylactic treatment following injury or in cases where a single broad-spectrum agent is not available. Similar to other broad-spectrum drugs, these agents allow the clinician to treat one infection while inhibiting secondary infection by another organism.

Antibiotic/corticosteroid combinations are also popular (Table 10-2). These allow simultaneous antibacterial coverage while decreasing the symptoms of inflammation. Disadvantages include increased toxicity and cost for the patient. These combinations are popular after ocular surgery, where there is also the risk of infection. These combined preparations will not be covered specifically in this text. However, the individual components are covered in their specific chapters.

Table 10-2
Selected Antibiotic/Steroid Ointments (Brand Names)

Bacitracin/Neomycin/Polymixin B/Hydrocortisone
Cortisporin
Coracin

Prednisolone Acetate/Gentamicin
Pred G SOP

Prednisolone/Sulfacetamide
Blephamide

Neomycin/Dexamethasone
Neodecadron

Tobramycin/Dexamethasone
Tobradex

Neomycin/Polymixin B/Dexamethasone
Ak-Trol
Dexacidin
Maxitrol

Selected Antibiotic/Steroid Solutions and Suspensions (Brand Names)

Neomycin/Hydocortisone
Cortisporin
Bactiocort

Fluorometholone/Sulfacetamide
FML-S

Oxytetracycline/Hydrocortisone
Terra-cortric

Neomycin/Hydrocortisone
Ak-Neo-Cort

Rhomycin/Prednisolone Acetate
Poly Pred

Gentamicin/Prednisolone Acetate
Pred-G

Neomycin/Dexamethasone sodium phosphate
Ak-Neo-Dex
Neo Decadron

Tobramycin/Dexamethasone
Dexacidin
Ak-Trol
Maxitrol
Dexasporin

Side Effects

The systemic effects and drug interactions of all antibiotics are too exhaustive to list. The potential for allergic, toxic, and other adverse reactions exists with all antimicrobial agents. Such responses are related to the specific drug chemistry, dosage, route of administration, age of the patient, and the patient's liver and kidney function. Specifics of individual ophthalmic drugs will be covered where applicable within the text. However, there are a few general conclusions that can be made about most antimicrobial therapies.

Allergy may result from any agent but is most commonly seen with use of the penicillins and sulfonamides. Such allergies can be very serious and life threatening, and they most often occur after injection and occur less commonly after oral administration. The likelihood of systemic reaction after topical administration of any drug is minimal and is lessened even more when punctal occlusion is employed.

Stomach upset and other gastrointestinal disturbances are very common after antibiotic therapy. This may be a consequence of direct irritation by the drug itself. The drug may also cause a reduction or overgrowth of the normal bacteria within the stomach and digestive system. These effects occur most often after oral administration of broad-spectrum antibiotics. The tetracycline antibiotics are well known for their frequent influence on the digestive tract.

Toxicity can result from higher doses or in lower dosages where the drug is not removed from the patient's system. For example, in some patients with decreased liver and/or kidney function, reduced excretion can lead to toxic drug levels building up rather quickly. Therefore, the liver and kidney function of patients, especially the elderly, must be evaluated before treatment. Toxicity can affect many different systems within the body. For example, auditory dysfunction can result from toxicity to systemically used aminoglycoside drugs.

Selected Antibacterials in Ophthalmic Practice

Bacitracin

Bacitracin is available alone or in combination drugs. As bacitracin alone, it comes only as an ointment (Ak-Tracin®). Though available OTC in other forms, ophthalmic preparations are by prescription only. Bacitracin is bacteriocidal mostly against gram-positive bacteria. Its advantages include minimal toxicity, few allergic reactions, and minimal resistance to it by the bacteria within its spectrum. However, given its limited spectrum, its major ophthalmic use is in the treatment of blepharitis.

Vancomycin

Vancomycin is a very potent bacteriocidal antibiotic. It is not marketed in topical ophthalmic form but is used orally and for injection. Vancomycin has very good gram-positive coverage. However, it is very toxic and is reserved for serious ocular infections where other drugs are not effective or cannot be used due to allergy.

Polymyxin B

Polymyxin B is another bacteriocidal drug that is not available alone as a topical ophthalmic product. It is very popular, however, in combination antibacterial formulations. The major value of polymyxin B is its effectiveness against *Pseudomonas aeruginosa*, a common cause of ocular infection. It is available as a powder in 20-ml vials, which is reconstituted as a solution for topical use or injection on the rare occasions where this is needed. Systemically, it is very toxic to the kidneys and nervous system; topically, there is minimal hypersensitivity.

Gramicidin

Gramicidin is an antibiotic with very little ophthalmologic use. It is bacteriocidal and has a spectrum of action similar to bacitracin, mostly against gram-positive bacteria. Because it can be formulated in solution and bacitracin cannot, its only beneficial use is as a replacement for bacitracin in certain antibiotic combinations.

Penicillins and Cephalosporins

Penicillins and cephalosporins are bacteriocidal agents occasionally used in ophthalmic practice in cases of lid, periorbital, and intraocular infections.

Examples of systemic penicillins include Penicillin G & V®, Dicloxacillin®, Amoxicillin®, Methacillin®, and Nafcillin®. As a group, penicillins have a broad spectrum of activity but are generally more effective against gram-positive organisms. However, they are unstable in solution and penetrate the cornea poorly. For these reasons, they are not available as topical ocular solutions or ointments. Another downside to the penicillins is a higher rate of allergic reaction. Up to 10% of patients will develop an allergy to penicillins, which can have serious consequences.

Cephalosporins (Keflex®, Keftab®, Ceclor®) are very similar to the penicillins and have generally the same spectrum and indications. They are commonly used in patients with allergies to penicillins. However, approximately 10% to 20% of patients with an allergy to penicillins will have a similar reaction to cephalosporins.

Historically, cephazolin (Ancef®, Kefzol®) has been a mainstay in the treatment of bacterial corneal ulcers. Though not marketed as an ophthalmic product, it is available for intravenous or subconjunctival injection. It may also be reconstituted into a fortified 0.5% solution for topical use. These fortified drops, however, are not preserved and expire after 4 days. Due to the inconvenience of preparing them, their short shelf life, and the effectiveness of the newer fluoroquinolones, the use of topical fortified cephazolin is becoming less popular.

The Aminoglycosides

There are 3 major aminoglycoside antibiotics available for ophthalmic use: neomycin, gentamicin, and tobramycin. They are very commonly used and are often the drug of choice in treating superficial ocular infections. All 3 have a relatively broad spectrum but are mostly active against gram-negative bacteria. Due to their widespread use, though, bacterial resistance to them is increasing. Further, if an organism is resistant to one aminoglycoside, it is usually resistant to the others as well. Systemic aminoglycoside use is not common due to its toxicity, which can result in auditory and vestibular dysfunction. Topical administration of aminoglycosides has not been linked to these adverse effects.

Neomycin

Neomycin has the broadest spectrum of the aminoglycoside therapeutics. It is available only in combination antibiotics and is very popular among general practitioners. Even so, neomycin has a major drawback. It is the most toxic of the aminoglycosides and possibly of all available topical antibiotics. At least 10% of patients will develop a hypersensitivity characterized by increased redness, swelling, and keratitis as early as several days after initiation of therapy. This can complicate the clinical picture. For this reason, and with better and less toxic drugs available, neomycin has limited value in today's ophthalmic practice.

Gentamicin

Available as gentamicin 0.3% ophthalmic ointment and solution (Garanycin®, Gentacidin®, Gentrasul®, Gentak®, Genoptic®), this broad-spectrum aminoglycoside has excellent gram-negative coverage. It is often the drug of choice as initial therapy of ocular surface infection. Less hypersensitivity occurs with gentamicin than with neomycin, but 50% of those allergic to neomycin will develop a reaction to gentamicin as well.

Tobramycin

Tobramycin is marketed as a 0.3% ophthalmic solution and ointment (Tobrex®, Defy®). Like the others in this class, it has a broad spectrum. It is slightly more effective than gentamicin, especially against *Pseudomonas aeruginosa*. Another benefit of tobramycin is that it is less toxic than gentamicin. Though bacteria are developing increased resistance to it, tobramycin is still the drug of choice for many ocular infections.

Tetracycline/Chlortetracycline

Tetracycline (Achromycin® 1% ophthalmic solution) and chlortetracycline (Aureomycin® 1% ophthalmic solution) are related bacteriostatic antibiotics. Both have a broad spectrum, with chlortetracycline having the edge against gram-negative bacteria. Because of their decreased relative effectiveness and increased bacterial resistance when compared to other available drugs, neither is the drug of choice in most situations. The tetracyclines are, however, effective in the treatment and prophylaxis of neonatal conjunctivitis and, combined with oral therapy, are useful in the treatment of ocular chlamydial infection.

Systemically, tetracycline and its relatives are also useful in the treatment of eyelid gland dysfunctions. The relatives of tetracycline are oxytetracycline (Teranycin®), doxycycline (Vibramycin®), and minocycline (Vectrin®, Minocin®). There are numerous downsides to systemic tetracycline therapy. First, it should not be used during pregnancy or in children younger than 8 years old because it may stain teeth and suppress bone development. Tetracyclines also affect the insulin requirements of diabetics and may reduce the effectiveness of oral contraceptives. Further, like a few other antibiotics, these therapeutics may increase the effects of blood-thinning medications. Tetracyclines may increase a patient's sensitivity to sunlight. As a general rule, they should not be taken with dairy products or antacids, which may decrease tetracycline's effectiveness.

Erythromycin

Erythromycin (AK-mycin®, Ilotycin®) belongs to a group called the macrolide antibiotics. Erythromycin may have bactericidal or bacteriostatic properties, depending on the specific organism. Its spectrum is broad but is more efficient against gram-positive bacteria. Erythromycin is rarely the drug of choice for any ocular infection. One reason for this is that it is only available as an ophthalmic ointment. On the positive side, it is relatively safe and nontoxic. For this reason, and its decent gram-positive spectrum, it is preferred by some clinicians for cases of chronic lid infection. Also, due to its safety, it is used instead of tetracycline for treatment of neonatal conjunctivitis or when the patient is allergic to tetracycline. Oral erythromycin is commonly used for infections in many parts of the body, including the eyelids and orbit. Again, however, it is usually reserved for cases where more effective antibiotics are contraindicated.

Overall, erythromycin is one of the safest antibiotics. Irritative effects, such as topical hypersensitivity, are infrequent. Nausea, diarrhea, and gastrointestinal upset may be experienced with oral administration. More serious complications, such as liver damage, are rare but possible. Lastly, some adverse drug interactions exist. One of these involves certain antihistamines. In general, oral antihistamine therapy and erythromycin should not be taken concurrently because fatal cardiac toxicity can result.

One other macrolide antibiotic is being used increasingly in ophthalmic practice. Azithromycin (Zithromax®) is proving effective in treating ocular chlamydial infection. Its advantage is that it can be administered orally as a single in-office dose rather than the traditional 21-day course of tetracycline.

Trimethoprim

Trimethoprim is available for ophthalmic use only in combination with polymyxin B (Polytrim®). Trimethoprim is another broad-spectrum antibiotic. Its spectrum does not cover *Pseudomonas aeruginosa*, so it is combined with polymyxin B to increase its effectiveness and uses. Adverse reactions are rare with Polytrim, and it has been shown safe in newborns and children. Given its safety and effectiveness—especially against *Haemophilus influenzae*, a common cause of eye and ear infections in children—Polytrim deserves primary consideration in the treatment of childhood conjunctivitis.

Sulfonamides

The sulfonamides are marketed as 4% sulfisoxazole (Gantrisin®) and as 10%, 15%, and 30% sodium sulfacetamide (AK-sulf®, Bleph 10®, Ocusulf®, Ophthacet®, Sulten-10®, Sulf-10®, Isopto Cetamide®, and Sodium Sulamyd®). They are available as both solution and ointment. They are also combined with steroids (Table 10-3).

Sulfonamides have been used in the treatment of bacterial infections for decades. Their spectrum is bacteriostatic against a wide range of gram-positive and gram-negative bacteria. Sulfonamides are still commonly used, especially in general practice and emergency rooms, but their popularity is declining. Their loss of popularity is mainly due to increasing resistance—reportedly up to 60% of some staph species, though this has recently been challenged. Sulfonamides also lose their effectiveness in the presence of heavy discharge, a byproduct of some bacterial infections. Lastly, they are incompatible with certain ocular anesthetics, particularly procaine and tetracaine.

Systemically, sulfonamide use has been replaced by other agents, with the exception of the treatment of toxoplasmosis. Allergic reactions resulting from sulfonamides are not uncommon, occurring with all routes of administration. Other effects reported with systemic sulfonamides use include blood disorders and transient myopia. Given their increasing resistance, limitations, and

Table 10-3
Selected Steroid/Sulfonamide Solutions and Suspensions

Combination	Trade Name
Sulfacetamide/Fluoromethalone	FML-S
Sulfacetamide/Prednisolone acetate	Blephamide
	Sulfacort
	Isopto Cetapred
	Ak-cide
	Ophtha P/S
	Metimyd
	Or-Toptic M
	Predsulfair
	Sulphrin
Sulfacetamide/Prednisolone phosphate	Vasocidin
	Optimyd

Steroid/Sulfonimide Ointments

Sulfacetamide/Prednisolone acetate	Blephamide SOP
	Cetapred
	Ak-cide
	Predsulfair
	Metimyd
	Vasocidin

Table 10-4
Flouroquinolones

Generic Name	Brand Name	Strength
Ciprofloxacin hydrochloride	Ciloxin	0.3%
Gatifloxacin	Zymar	0.3%
Levofloxacin	Iquix	1.5%
	Quixin	0.5%
Moxifloxacin	Vigamox	0.5%
Ofloxacin	Oculflox	0.3%

the availability of more effective therapeutics, the sulfonamides are now a poor choice in most instances of ocular bacterial infections.

Fluoroquinolones

The fluoroquinolone group consists of several generational drugs (Table 10-4) (Note: Each version of a drug is considered a "generation." If a drug changes formulation, as we have seen with the fluorquinolones, the first version of the molecule is considered the first generation, and so on.) These new antibiotics have quickly established themselves as the "top gun" of ophthalmic antibacterial drugs most commonly used today. The fluoroquinolones are extremely effective bacteriocidal drugs, having a broad spectrum with increased effectiveness against gram-negative pathogens. They have several advantages over other antimicrobials. First, they have a very low corneal toxicity, though ciprofloxacin has been shown to form an occasional white precipitate in courses of treatment of corneal ulcers. Secondly, these therapeutics have a very rapid kill rate, which not only increases their effectiveness but allows little time for bacteria to acquire resistance, a rarity with these agents. Lastly, they have very good corneal penetration. Ofloxacin has been shown to have greater aqueous concentration than the others, but it is questionable whether this is clinically significant. Adverse reactions are rare with topical use. However, safety and efficacy in children younger than 12 and nursing mothers has not been established.

Only ciprofloxacin and ofloxacin are approved by the FDA for the treatment of corneal ulcers. Since their arrival, they are replacing the time-tested use of fortified tobramycin and cefazolin for this application because recent studies have shown equal or better efficacy. Fluoroquinolones are also less expensive, more convenient, and have a longer shelf life than the fortified antibiotics. Cultures and sensitivity testing should be done on all corneal ulcers to determine which drugs will be most effective in the eradication of the causative bacteria.

There is concern that with increasing popularity will come increased resistance. Over time, this may diminish the effectiveness of the powerful therapeutics. Therefore, we reserve the use of these agents for cases of severe infection or where sight is threatened. (See Table 10-4 for a list of flouroquinolones.)

Antiviral Therapy

OphT

Viruses are the smallest of all the infectious agents. They work by invading and taking charge of a cell's genetic and reproductive machinery. They use their newly acquired machinery to reproduce new viruses, which then repeat the process again. Thankfully, this highly effective invasion is stopped by our own immune system, and most viral infections are acute and self-limiting. Occasionally, however, a virus can invade and set up camp in a dormant or latent state. The latent state protects the virus from the immune system. Then, on occasion, the virus "awakens," and an acute viral infection begins. The active virus can be destroyed, but the latent one remains, waiting for another time to reactivate. Recurrences of these viral infections can be common, especially in immunocompromised patients who lack the defenses to fight them off.

OphA

There are very few effective antiviral drugs because it is difficult to formulate a drug that eradicates the virus from the cells without also killing the cells themselves. The currently available antiviral therapeutics are mostly effective in treating the herpes virus, of which there are 4 main types. The first is the herpes simplex virus (the cause of cold sores), genital herpes, and herpes simplex keratitis. The second is the varicella zoster virus, the virus causing chicken pox and shingles. The third variety is the Epstein-Barr virus, which causes mononucleosis. Last, is the cytomegalovirus, a common infectious agent in AIDS patients.

There are 3 main antiviral therapeutics for topical ophthalmic use: idoxuridine, vidarabine, and trifluridine. Three others—ganciclovir, foscarnet, and acyclovir—will also be discussed briefly.

Idoxuridine

Idoxuridine is available as 0.1% ophthalmic solution under the name Herplex®. It is indicated for use in treatment of herpes simplex keratitis. Ocularly, this agent is relatively safe, though corneal toxicity can arise if used for prolonged periods. For this reason, it is advised that it not be used for more than 21 days. Systemic idoxuridine is very toxic and is not used. Idoxuridine was the original antiviral developed and has since been surpassed in effectiveness by other agents.

Vidarabine

Vidarabine is also used in the treatment of herpes simplex keratitis infection as an intravenous solution. The advantages of vidarabine are that it is less toxic than idoxuridine and is usually effective in instances where idoxuridine is not. However, both have largely been replaced by succeeding antivirals.

Trifluridine

Trifluridine 1% ophthalmic solution (Viroptic®) is without exception the drug of choice for epithelial keratitis secondary to herpes simplex. When used every 2 hours, or 9 times daily, it is superior to either vidarabine or idoxuridine. Trifluridine has better penetration, is more effective, and exhibits no cross resistance to its counterparts. Corneal toxicity can develop over time, and duration of therapy should normally not exceed 21 days. It is also a very expensive drug.

Ganciclovir and Foscarnet

Two very potent antiviral drugs, ganciclovir and foscarnet, are experiencing widespread use in the treatment of cytomegalovirus retinitis. This retinal infection is potentially blinding and is normally seen in immunocompromised AIDS patients. Used alone or together, both drugs have been shown to significantly delay the progress and recurrence of cytomegalovirus retinitis. However, neither cures the disease. Ganciclovir (Cytovene®) can be used orally, intravenously, or can be implanted into the vitreous of the affected eye. The implant is marketed as Vitrasert®. The Vitrasert is implanted into the affected eye, where the ganciclovir is released locally to the site of infection. Blurred vision results, lasting several weeks. Over time, the store of ganciclovir is depleted. The insert can be removed 6 to 8 months later. Foscarnet is only available as a solution for intravenous use (Foscavir®).

When either drug is used for intravenous therapy, an initial (induction) dosage is started 2 to 3 times daily for up to 3 weeks, then once daily thereafter. Toxicity with oral or intravenous use is high. Ganciclovir can cause bone marrow suppression and decreased numbers of white blood cells. Foscarnet has no severe bone marrow suppression, but kidney impairment and seizures have resulted from its use. The Vitrasert, because of its local action, does not have these associated side effects to the same degree as the systemic routes of administration. The drawback to vitreal insert is that bilateral treatment may be necessary, requiring 2 procedures for implantation.

Acyclovir

The use of oral acyclovir (Zovirax®) has proven effective in the treatment of both ocular and nonocular manifestation of herpes simplex virus and varicella zoster virus. The usual regimen for herpes simplex virus is 400 mg 5 times daily. Unlike most oral anti-infectives, acyclovir is able to reach therapeutic levels in the tears and aqueous. Though shown effective when used alone, it is usually paired with topical trifluridine for better action. For varicella zoster infections, the dosage is increased to 800 mg 5 times daily. Even at these concentrations, acyclovir is remarkably nontoxic systemically, normally causing only mild stomach upset on occasion. Zovirax is available as 200, 400, and 800 mg tablets. It can also be found as a 5% dermatologic ointment for treatment of skin lesions. Though shown effective in studies, no topical ophthalmic ointment is available in the United States.

Famcyclovir

Famcyclovir (Famvir®) is very similar to acyclovir; however, famcyclovir is not specifically indicated for treatment of ophthalmic manifestations of shingles. Both acyclovir and famcyclovir are activated by virally affected cells only, and healthy cells remain unaffected. For this reason, both have a very low toxicity. The benefit of famcyclovir versus acyclovir is that famcyclovir has longer activity, which means it can be used on a regimen of 500 mg 3 times daily. However, because famcyclovir was only recently approved in 1994, acyclovir remains the primary therapeutic in the treatment of herpes zoster virus.

Valacyclovir

Valacyclovir (Valtrex®) is a newer generation antiviral medication. It is given as an oral treatment for Herpes simplex virus as well as Herpes zoster. When administered, it converts to acyclovir (see previous page).

Antifungal Therapy

Fungal infections are caused by plantlike microorganisms. These infections can be devastating to the eye and a challenge to the practitioner who encounters them. Luckily, only a few hundred cases occur in the United States every year. However, their numbers are increasing. Natamycin (Natacyn®) is currently the only approved topical antifungal therapeutic for ophthalmic use. Both fungicidal and nontoxic to the cornea, it is effective against many different types of fungi. Marketed as a 5% suspension, it is usually prescribed every 1 or 2 hours for 2 to 3 weeks. However, if this fails to bring improvement in 7 to 10 days, the infectious organism is likely unaffected by natamycin. In cases where natamycin is ineffective, several other systemic antifungals (sometimes converted to solutions), such as fluconazole (Diflucan®), idraconazole (Sporanox®), amphotericin B, miconazole, ketoconazole (Nizoral®), and flucytosine, have been used with varied success.

Bibliography

Bartlett JD, Jaanus SD, eds. *Clinical Ocular Pharmacology*. 2nd ed. Stoneham, Mass: Butterworths; 1988.

Biro S. FDA approves oral gancyclovir as CMV retinitis preventative. *Primary Care Optometry News.* 1996;1(1):36-37.

Bohigian GM. *Handbook of Extended Diseases of the Eye*. 2nd ed. St. Louis, Mo: DXC Medical Publishing Assoc; 1980.

Catania LJ. *Primary Care of the Anterior Segment*. East Norwalk, Conn: Appleton and Lange; 1988.

Ellis PP. *Ocular Therapeutics and Pharmacology*. 6th ed. St. Louis, Mo: CV Mosby; 1981.

Kuman V, Cotram RS, Robbins SL. *Basic Pathology*. 5th ed. Philadelphia, Pa: WB Saunders; 1992.

Marielo EN. *Human Anatomy & Physiology*. Redwood City, Calif: Benjamin/Cummings Publishing; 1989.

Melton R, Thomas R. 4th Annual guide to therapeutic drugs. *Optometic Management:* Norwalk Conn.; May 1995.

Moses RA, Hart W Jr. *Adler's Physiology of the Eye: Clinical Application* 8th ed. St. Louis, Mo: CV Mosby; 1987.

Onofrey BE, ed. *Clinical Optometrics Pharmacology & Therapeutics*. Philadelphia, Pa: JB Lippincott; 1992.

Ophthalmic Drug Facts. St. Louis, Mo: JB Lippincott; 1990.

PDR for Ophthalmology. 23rd ed. Montvale, NJ: Medical Economics; 1995.

Silverman HM, ed. *The Pill Book.* 6th ed. New York, NY: Bantam Books; 1994.

Stephenson M. FDA panel recommends implant for approval. *Primary Care Optometry News.* 1996;1(1):37.

Chapter 11

Antiglaucoma Agents

- Glaucoma treatment is targeted to decrease the IOP in order to reduce or stop further optic nerve damage and visual field loss. This is done pharmacologically by decreasing aqueous production or increasing outflow.

- Although laser and filtering surgery has advanced, retiring many traditional drugs, pharmacologic management is still the primary step in the treatment of glaucoma.

- Beta blockers have long been the drug of choice in glaucoma management. However, newer medications, such as topical carbonic anhydrase inhibitors and prostaglandin analogues, have replaced them.

- Glaucoma therapy involves treating the patient, not just the disease. Factors relating to patient compliance, lifestyle, systemic heath, as well as the expense of therapy must always be considered when determining the appropriate course of action.

An Overview

Glaucoma is a neurodegenerative disease that classically presents with a triad of elevated IOP, optic nerve damage, and constriction of the peripheral visual field. The medical management of glaucoma is to decrease IOP in order to halt or slow the progression of optic nerve and visual field loss.

The ciliary body produces a fluid called aqueous. The aqueous flows from the ciliary body and exits through a "drain" called the trabecular meshwork, located in the anterior chamber angle. Aqueous nourishes the eye's interior and creates pressure inside the eye. Elevated IOP results when aqueous is produced faster than it can be drained. If this pressure is elevated, optic nerve and visual field damage can result. Using the common analogy of a sink, either the faucet is turned up too high or the drainpipe is clogged. Pharmaceuticals have been developed with the purpose of reducing aqueous production or increasing drainage.

Antiglaucoma medications are often classified according to their action on the autonomic nervous system. (A basic understanding of the autonomic nervous system is given in Chapter 3.) By pharmacologically stimulating or inhibiting the neurotransmitter-receptor link at specific sites within the eye, the balance between fluid production and outflow can be altered. The parasympathetic system has 2 types of receptors: nicotinic and muscarinic. Muscarinic receptors are present in the iris, ciliary body, and trabecular meshwork. Stimulation of these receptors in the iris causes miosis. In the ciliary body, there is stimulation of certain fibers, which creates a mechanical pulling effect, opening the trabecular meshwork and increasing aqueous drainage. Muscarinic receptors in the trabecular meshwork may also play a role in increased aqueous outflow.

The sympathetic (or adrenergic) nervous system relies on different receptors, of which there are 4 types: alpha$_1$, alpha$_2$, beta$_1$, and beta$_2$. Stimulation of alpha receptors in the iris causes mydriasis while stimulation of the same receptors in the ciliary body results in decreased aqueous production. Basically, most beta receptors oppose the alpha receptor actions. When beta receptors within the ciliary body are activated, there is an increased aqueous flow. Beta receptors located in the trabecular meshwork increase drainage. Though not completely understood, stimulation of the alpha$_2$ receptors has an inhibitory effect on sympathetic neurotransmitter (norepinephrine) release. With less norepinephrine released, there is possibly less stimulation of the beta receptors and an overall decreased aqueous production.

Direct-Acting Adrenergic Drugs

Epinephrine Compounds

Epinephrine is a naturally occurring substance in our bodies. Though it has been used in the treatment of glaucoma for many years, its mechanism is still not fully understood. It has an effect on all alpha and beta receptors. Most likely, it stimulates contraction of blood vessels in the ciliary body, thus reducing aqueous formation. It has also been shown to increase outflow. Whatever its action, it is a fairly weak-acting antiglaucoma medication. Historically, its use was mainly as an additive to pilocarpine and beta blockers. Much more effective agents are now available, and the use of epinephrine is declining. Available in 0.5%, 1%, and 2% (Epifrin®, Epitrate®, Glaucon®, Eppy/N®, Epinal®), it is normally used twice a day. To aid in recognition and patient compliance, epinephrine is usually marketed in a brown bottle or a red-labeled bottle with a white

What the Patient Needs to Know

- Glaucoma is a lifelong disease. It is not cured like an infection. Drops must be taken every day.

- Never stop medication unless advised to do so by your physician. Glaucoma causes damage to the eye even if you "feel" fine. Always return for your scheduled pressure checks.

- Some drops sting when you put them in. However, if drops cause eyes to sting for prolonged periods, notify your doctor.

- Gels and ointments should be the last medication put in the eye if a series of medications is used.

- Wait a minimum of 5 minutes between drops if multiple drops are used.

- Gels and ointments blur vision. Putting them in just before sleeping reduces this inconvenience.

- After using glaucoma drops, close your eyes and gently press your forefinger against the corner of your eye, next to the nose. This seals off the tear-drainage system, keeping the medication on the eye. It also helps reduce the chances of the drug entering your body system, thereby decreasing side effects.

- Follow the doctor's directions exactly.

- Keep a schedule of when you take your medication. This is helpful to the doctor.

- Have others remind you to take your medication. Have someone else put the medicine in for you if you have a hard time.

- To help you remember to use your medicine and to make things handy, keep a bottle of drops in the places where you usually are when drop-time rolls around. For example, keep a bottle at home, one in your desk at work, one in your workshop, etc.

- Does not stop medication because of the cost. Ask your doctor about less costly alternatives.

- Taking more than the prescribed dose will not help. It may hurt and is more expensive.

- Take your drops on schedule even when you have an appointment for a pressure check.

- Never run out of medication. Be sure to get refills before the bottle or tube is empty. A weekend without medication is a weekend where your pressure runs high. That could mean a weekend where your optic nerve is irreparably damaged.

- For proper drop control, some medications are packaged in bottles that are larger than necessary, giving the appearance of being half-full when purchased. This is not a manufacturing error. The amount of drug in the container is the proper amount.

- Advise your physician if redness, swelling, or scaling of the eyelids occurs because this may indicate a sensitivity to the medication.

Note: A few patient education notes regarding selected medications are found at the end of this chapter. Every patient should be advised about the possible side effects of every new drug he or she is given.

cap. A combination of 1% epinephrine and pilocarpine is available as E-Pilo®. This drug is designated by the numbers 1 through 6, the numbers referring to the percentage of pilocarpine.

Dipivefrin 0.1% (Propine®) is a pro drug of epinephrine. It crosses the cornea more easily than epinephrine and is converted into epinephrine in the eye. Its indications and use are the same as epinephrine. Dipivefrin is packaged with a purple cap.

Both drugs arouse the sympathetic system. They should be used with caution in the presence of cardiovascular disease, diabetes, hyperthyroidism, or asthma. Overall, due to its formulation, dipivefrin is safer than epinephrine, but the same relative warnings exist. Ocularly, both are quite uncomfortable after instilling and may cause conjunctival redness. Over time, hypersensitivity is not uncommon, and pigmented spots, called adrenochrome deposits, may be seen in the conjunctiva.

Alpha$_2$ Adrenergic Agonists

Though not completely understood, alpha$_2$ adrenergic agonists bind with alpha$_2$ receptors and decrease aqueous production.

Apraclonidine

Until very recently, apraclonidine (Iopidine®) was the only available alpha$_2$ agonist. It is available in 0.5% and 1.0% solutions. The 1.0% solution can be used pre- and postsurgically to control "pressure spikes," as rapid elevation in IOP is particularly common after laser procedures. Normally, 1 drop is instilled into the preoperative eye 1 hour before surgery and another immediately following the procedure.

The 0.5% solution is used for short-term adjunctive glaucoma therapy when multiple medications are being used. Use of this medication for chronic IOP control has little success. Though useful in the short term, chronic use usually fails, with more than 50% of patients experiencing decreased effectiveness after a few months. Close monitoring is necessary. Also, a large number of patients (conservatively reported at 75%) will develop allergic reactions. Like any drug affecting the nervous system, risks are possible. However, apraclonidine is one of the safest pharmaceuticals in the glaucoma arsenal. Systemic side effects are rare, but dry mouth, a bad taste, and systemic hypotension are occasionally noticed. For adjunctive therapy, apraclonidine is used 3 times daily.

Brimonidine

Brimonidine (Alphagan®) is the latest addition to this class of the antiglaucoma armamentarium. It is also an alpha adrenergic agonist. Whereas apraclonidine generally affects both alpha and alpha$_2$ receptors, brimonidine is a highly selective alpha$_2$ adrenergic agonist. This selectivity results in fewer side effects when compared to apraclonidine. Brimonidine causes little or no acceleration of the breathing rate and has a low incidence of allergic response (about 7%).

Brimonidine is reported to have a dual mechanism of action, both decreasing aqueous production and increasing aqueous outflow. This dual nature means that brimonidine can probably be used along with other pressure lowering agents, although further study is needed in this area. Brimonidine is also relatively fast acting, with effects shown within the first hour after administration. It may, therefore, be a good choice for reduction of pressure spikes after intraocular surgery.

Though comparative studies have shown little difference in effect between 2 or 3 times a day dosing, the manufacturer recommends 3 times daily. Alphagan is packaged in a container with a purple cap.

Brimonidine has the potential to challenge or supplant traditional first-line therapies. Studies show similar efficacy as the time-honored timolol maleate. However, unlike beta blockers, there are no contraindications in patients with pulmonary disease. Furthermore, brimonidine does not decrease the heart rate. Systemic hypotension is a concern with the alpha adrenergic agonists, though it is not commonly seen. Dryness of the mouth has commonly been reported with the use of brimonidine, but ocular dryness is less pronounced than with topical carbonic anhydrase inhibitors. This is due in part to brimonidine's formulation with a polyvinyl alcohol, a common component in artificial tears.

Alphagan, like the other recently introduced medications Trusopt® and Xalatan®, has the potential to change the traditional face of glaucoma treatment. However, time will be the judge of whether or not the promise and potential of these agents are fulfilled.

Adrenergic Antagonists (Beta Blockers)

`OphT`

The adrenergic antagonists are commonly referred to as beta blockers. Their action is to block the activity caused by stimulation of the adrenergic beta receptors. When stimulated, these receptors are responsible for increasing aqueous production. Thus, when blocked, aqueous production is reduced. Since their introduction in the late 1970s, use of the beta blockers has grown to become the most frequently prescribed drug for glaucoma therapy. These adrenergic antagonistic therapeutics are safely used in combination with epinephrine compounds, miotics, and carbonic anhydrase inhibitors when multiple medications are needed.

With one exception, beta blockers act equally on both beta and beta$_2$ receptors. Beta$_2$ receptors are present in both the heart and lungs. Stimulation of these causes decreased heart rate and decreased breathing. As a result, beta blockers are generally contraindicated in patients with cardiovascular and respiratory disease, particularly asthma and chronic obstructive pulmonary disease (COPD). Baseline blood pressure and heart rate are recommended before therapy when a beta blocker is instituted, and monitoring is recommended thereafter. Another commonly reported systemic effect is depression.

Ocularly, the beta blockers cause irritation in fewer than half of those using them. Decreased corneal sensation is also reported, though it is uncommon. Most beta blockers are prescribed for use twice a day. They all have yellow or light blue caps.

Timolol

Timolol maleate (Timoptic®) was the first ophthalmic beta blocker available. In addition to 0.25% and 0.5% solutions, 2 other formulations are marketed. The first is Timoptic in Ocudose® unit dose dispensers. Supplied in boxes of 60, it is preservative-free for patients with a history of preservative sensitivity. Recently, Timoptic has also been redesigned into a gel-forming solution (Timoptic XE®) in the same 2 concentrations. Timoptic XE has an increased contact time with the eye and, thus, provides longer absorption. This allows it to be used once daily. The disadvantage of the gel-forming solution is that it blurs the vision for some time after instillation. This drawback can be eliminated if it is administered before going to sleep each night. While research suggests an increased effect if administered in the morning, this increased effect is minimal, and the advantage of evening administration outweighs this small increase in effectiveness.

Another addition to the timolol family is timolol hemihydrate (Betamol®), available in 0.25% and 0.5% concentrations. Studies show similar results with this "new drug" when compared to the traditional timolol maleate solutions. Though it has no advantage over timolol maleate in its ability to lower IOP the cost to the patient is somewhat lower. This decreased cost may lead to increased compliance.

Levobunolol

Levobunolol 0.5% (Betagan®) is virtually identical in concentrations and effect to the timolol drugs, except that is has been approved for once daily administration. However, while some patients do receive adequate IOP control with once-a-day usage, most patients require instillation twice a day for proper IOP reduction. Levobunolol is less expensive than Timoptic XE (the only other "once daily" beta blocker). However, the results with Timoptic XE on this schedule are significantly better. The 0.25% concentration of levobunolol must be used twice daily.

Metipranolol

Metipranolol (Optipranolol® 0.3%) is another nonspecific beta receptor antagonist. Its effects are comparable to timolol 0.25%. The one true advantage of this product is that it is considerably less expensive than all other beta blockers. However, there is some concern because of implications of the role of metapranolol in cases of severe anterior segment inflammation. This topic is still being debated. Nonetheless, Optipranolol is still a viable choice when a beta blocker is needed and cost is a major concern.

Carteolol

Carteolol HCl 1% ophthalmic solution (Ocupress®) is a unique beta blocker. Although its effect is similar to timolol 0.5%, it possesses some qualities that may make it a safer choice. First, it has a unique makeup that impedes its crossing of the blood-brain barrier. This reduces the risk of central nervous system effects, such as depression, not altogether uncommon with beta blockers. Second, carteolol has intrinsic sympathomimetic activity (ISA). Whereas other nonselective beta blockers tend to fully block all beta receptor sites, carteolol, with its ISA, seems to have a partial or incomplete blocking potential. Decreased systemic side effects may be the result. Lastly, other nonselective beta blockers have been shown to adversely affect fatty substances within the blood (lipids) and may also decrease blood supply to the optic nerve through vasoconstriction. Carteolol may have less of a negative impact on these than more traditional beta blockers.

Betaxolol

Betaxolol is available in a 0.5% solution (Betoptic®) and a 0.25% suspension (Betoptic-S®). Due to its formulation, Betoptic-S is equivalent in effect to Betoptic, though it is a smaller concentration and is associated with fewer side effects. Both are used twice daily.

Betaxolol is different from all other beta blockers in that it has selective activity. Traditional beta blockers affect beta and $beta_2$ receptors equally. Betaxolol has much greater affinity for beta receptors only, though it is still minimally active at $beta_2$ receptor sites. The adverse cardiopulmonary effects associated with nonselective beta blockers are mostly due to beta$_2$ receptor stimulation. Thus, there are fewer of these associated risks with betaxolol, which is relatively safer for patients with heart or lung disease. However, the same potential risks still exist, and other agents are usually better first-choice alternatives for these patients due to their decreased cardiopulmonary risks.

Cholinergics (Miotics)

OphT

Srg

Cholinergic agents mimic the actions of the parasympathetic nervous system. One effect of the parasympathetic response is contraction of the iris sphincter, causing the pupil to get smaller (miosis). For this reason, the cholinergic drugs are commonly referred to as miotics. All miotics are additive to beta blockers and sympathomimetic agents. They may be direct acting or indirect acting.

The direct-acting agents decrease IOP by increasing the flow of aqueous out of the eye. When the muscarinic receptors in the ciliary body are stimulated, certain fibers of the ciliary body contract. This mechanically opens the drainage system of the trabecular meshwork and increases aqueous outflow. Pilocarpine and carbachol are the 2 direct-acting cholinergics currently available, though less commonly used today.

The indirect-acting cholinergics act in a slightly different way. Also known as anticholinesterase drugs, they work by preventing the "clean up" of the neurotransmitter at the receptor site. The neurotransmitter can then remain at the site and have a prolonged effect. Anticholinesterase drugs are classified as reversible or irreversible. If the drug is reversible, it has a short action (several hours). Irreversible anticholinesterase drugs have a prolonged action, sometimes lasting up to several days. There are 4 available anticholinesterase therapeutics. Physostigmine and demercarium bromide are reversible, while echothiophate iodine and isoflurophate are irreversible.

Aside from glaucoma treatment, the miotic drugs are also used in cases of overcorrection (hyperopia) after refractive surgery. The agents most commonly used for this are pilocarpine and echothiophate iodine. Finally, though their miotic property can help to reverse the action of mydriatic drops, this is not recommended because it may induce an acute angle-closure glaucoma attack.

Ocular side effects are reported frequently with cholinergic therapy. Though true allergic reactions are rare, these agents commonly sting on instillation. They also cause brow ache, headache, accommodative spasm, and induced myopia. These effects are more pronounced in younger patients. While these problems may be substantial when therapy is first instituted, they decrease over time.

The miotic nature of these drugs must be also be taken into account. In patients with cataracts, miosis can markedly decrease vision. Historically, miotics have been said to increase the risk of retinal detachment and cataracts, though this has not been conclusively established. Systemic adverse effects are similar with all cholinergic drugs and include sweating, salivation, stomach and digestive upset, and decreased heart rate. Miotic therapy has proven efficacy and is an inexpensive option. However, with the possible exception of the gel and sustained-release systems (to be discussed shortly), miotic therapy is usually associated with poor compliance—a result of patient discomfort and the frequent administration required (often 4 times a day).

Direct-Acting Cholinergics

Pilocarpine

Pilocarpine is the drug of choice when miotic therapy is indicated in the treatment of glaucoma. It is available in solution concentrations ranging from 0.25% to 10% (Isoptocarpine®, Pilagan®, Pilocar®, Piloptic®, Pilostat®, Adsorbocarpine®, Alcarpine®). The 1% to 4% concentrations are most commonly used. Higher concentration may have additional value, but side effects increase; these concentrations are sometimes more valuable in dark-eyed patients because pilocarpine tends to have a decreased effect in these patients. Dosage is usually 4 times daily, though it may be used as little as once or as often as 6 times per day, depending on the desired effect.

Pilocarpine is also available as a 4% gel (Pilopine HS®) to be administered nightly. The advantages are increased patient compliance and patient comfort. By applying the gel at bedtime, the adverse effects of headache, brow ache, and accommodative spasm will likely occur when the patient is asleep.

A pilocarpine time-released delivery system is also available. Marketed as Ocusert®, it is a thin wafer-shaped disk that is placed in the inferior conjunctival cul-de-sac. The wafer is replaced weekly. It is available in 2 strengths: Ocusert pilo-20 (equivalent to 2%) and Ocusert pilo-40 (equivalent to 4%).

Carbachol

Carbachol (Isopto Carbachol®) is available in 0.75%, 1.5%, 2.25%, and 3.0% concentrations. It is somewhat stronger than pilocarpine, and its miotic-related ocular side effects are more pronounced. Further, it is more toxic to the cornea and does not penetrate as well. The use of carbachol is reserved for patients who are not getting adequate pressure control from pilocarpine. Today, it is rarely prescribed, though many patients remain well controlled with carbachol and continue its use. Administration is 3 times daily.

Intraocular Agents

Two direct-acting cholinergic agents are available for intraocular administration during surgery. Acetylcholine (Michol-E®) and carbachol 0.1% (Miostat®) are used to induce miosis, particularly during some cataract surgeries. Miostat has also recently been indicated for the control of IOP increases in the 24 hours immediately following cataract surgery.

Indirect-Acting Cholinergics (Acetylcholinesterase Agents)

Physostigmine (Eserine)

Physostigmine (Isoptoeserine®) is the weakest of the cholinesterase inhibitors. Its only indication is for glaucoma treatment when other miotics have failed. Solutions of 0.25% and 0.5% are available for use up to 4 times daily. A 0.25% ointment is also on the market. Physostigmine is rarely used anymore. A physostigmine/pilocarpine combination is available; however, it possesses no better action than either drug alone and is, therefore, not often recommended.

Demercarium Bromide, Echothiophate Iodine, Isoflurophate

These 3 agents are indicated for, but rarely used in, the treatment of glaucoma. Their potent effect and long action makes them more useful in the diagnosis and treatment of accommodative esotropia. Echothiophate is sometimes valuable in treating over-correction after refractive surgery.

Demercarium bromide (Humorsol®) solution is available in 0.125% and 0.25% concentrations. Echothiophate iodine (Phospholine Iodine®) is available as a powder for reconstitution into 0.06%, 0.03%, 0.125%, and 0.25% concentrations. Isoflurophate (Floropryl®) is only available as 0.025% ophthalmic ointment.

All 3 may induce serious ocular and systemic side effects and may be used only when all other glaucoma medications and surgery fail. Their ocular and systemic side effects are similar to, but more pronounced than, those seen with miotics such as pilocarpine. Rare cases of iris cyst or lens opacity formation as well as retinal detachment have been reported. These drugs still maintain value in management of other specific ocular conditions.

Carbonic Anhydrase Inhibitors

`OphT`

Carbonic anhydrase is a critical enzyme in the physiologic pathway of aqueous production. When inhibited, there is a decrease in aqueous production and a resultant drop in IOP.

Traditionally, carbonic anhydrase inhibitors (CAIs) have been administered orally. These agents are well absorbed and very effective, but they are poorly tolerated long-term due to their adverse effects. About 50% of patients will need to discontinue systemic CAI therapy within several months.

Common systemic effects are depression, stomach discomfort, tingling of the extremities, kidney stones, and impotence. A substantial metallic, chalky taste is also common. The tingling of the extremities is so pronounced that it has been suggested that you can judge a patient's compliance by asking if this sensation is present. Ocular effects with systemic therapy are rare. All CAIs, topical or systemic, are contraindicated in patients with sulfonamide allergies, severe kidney or heart diseases, and adrenocortical insufficiency.

Topical Carbonic Anhydrase Inhibitors

Dorzolamide

Recently, dorzolamide 2.0% (Trusopt®) emerged as the first topical CAI for the treatment of glaucoma. The effectiveness of oral CAIs is well known, but their adverse reactions severely limit their use. A topical CAI, having few of those adverse effects, is a long-awaited and very welcome addition to the antiglaucoma arsenal. The most common side effect of this topical CAI is ocular irritation and bitter taste. Its pressure-lowering effects are additive to beta blockers.

Dorzolamide is approved for administration 3 times daily. However, twice-a-day administration has been investigated and found effective, though the IOP-lowering effect is reduced by about 20%. Thus, in many cases, twice-a-day administration is often first initiated and increased to 3 times a day if additional IOP control is necessary. Dorzolamide may have a decreased effect in patients with darkly pigmented irises, and use 3 times a day may be necessary in these individuals.

Systemic Carbonic Anhydrase Inhibitors

Acetazolamide

Acetazolamide is available as 125 and 250 mg tablets (Diamox®, AK-zol®, Diazamide®). The usual dosage is 250 mg to 1 g in divided doses over 24 hours. Acetazolamide is also available as a 500 mg sustained-release capsule (Diamox Sequels®) providing 18 to 24 hours of action, compared to 8 to 12 for the tablets. The recommended dosage is 1 capsule twice daily. Acetazolamide is also available as Diamox parenteral 500 mg. This is a sterile powder that is reconstituted before injection. It is indicated for rapid reduction of IOP and for use before or during ocular surgery, when oral medication cannot be taken.

For treatment of primary open-angle glaucoma, acetazolamide is reserved for patients whose pressure is not controlled with methazolamide. Acetazolamide has more adverse effects than methazolamide, so it is the second choice. However, acetazolamide is the preferred agent in cases of acute angle-closure glaucoma due to its greater IOP-lowering effect.

Methazolamide

Methazolamide (Neptazane®, Glauctabs®, MZM®) is available in 25 or 50 mg tablets. Usual dosage is 25 mg twice daily but may be increased to a maximum of 50 mg 3 times daily. Clinically significant pressure reduction with more than 100 mg daily is questionable, and side effects increase. Methazolamide is the preferred choice when a systemic CAI is indicated in glaucoma therapy. This preference is due to decreased systemic side effects, particularly kidney stones.

Dichlorphenamide

Dichlorphenamide 50 mg (Dramadine®) is a very potent CAI and has the greatest incidence of unwanted effects. Therefore, it is used only when the other drugs in this class fail to adequately control the IOP. Some patients unable to take acetazolamide and methazolamide have been tolerant of dichlorphenamide. The patients who can tolerate this drug are few, and the use of this agent is exceedingly rare. Administration is 100 mg every 2 hours until the desired effect is obtained, then reduction to a maintenance level of 25 to 50 mg up to 3 times daily.

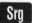

Hyperosmotics

Systemic hyperosmotics quickly reduce IOP by drawing aqueous out of the eye. Their most common use in ophthalmology is in cases of acute angle-closure glaucoma.

The effect of these drugs comes from their ability to increase the concentration of particles in the blood plasma. The concentration of particles rises and is no longer in equilibrium with that of water. Water will move out of the body tissues and into the plasma to restore this equilibrium. As fluid leaves the eye and moves into the plasma, the IOP decreases.

As excess fluid moves out of the body, tissues can dehydrate, resulting in thirst, headache, and disorientation. Patients complaining of thirst during treatment should not be given a drink if at all possible because this will counteract the effect. The increased fluid in the bloodstream can also result in cardiac problems. Systemic hyperosmotics are contraindicated in patients suffering from severe kidney or heart disease. They are also not indicated for chronic IOP control. Oral hyperosmotics are extremely sweet, and this may induce nausea or vomiting. It is suggested that serving them chilled, over ice while sipped through a straw, may make them more tolerable.

Table 11-1 Prostaglandins		
Generic Name	**Brand Name**	**Strength**
Bimatoprost	Lumigan	0.03%
Latanoprost	Xalatan	0.005%
Travoprost	Travatan	0.004%
Unoprostone	Rescula	0.15%

Glycerin (Glycerol)

Glycerin (Osmoglyn® 50%) is the first of the 2 oral hyperosmotics. The dosage is based on the weight of the patient, approximately 2 ml to 3 ml per kilogram of body weight. For the average sized adult, this is approximately 6 oz. Osmoglyn comes plain or lime-flavored. Glycerin is not recommended for use in diabetic patients. Absorbed through the stomach, it is metabolized by the body, resulting in a heavy caloric load. This can lead to hyperglycemia and other adverse effects. A better choice in diabetic patients is isosorbide.

Isosorbide

Isosorbide oral solution (Ismotic® 45%), unlike glycerol, is not metabolized and is, therefore, safer in diabetic patients. Otherwise, its effects are similar to glycerol. The flavor of this brown solution is described as vanilla mint. Dosage is 1.5 g per kilogram, or about 1.5 ml per pound, of body weight.

Intravenous Hyperosmotics

Mannitol

Mannitol (Osmitrol®) is the only systemic hyperosmotic for intravenous use. It can be used in both the treatment of acute angle-closure glaucoma or before ocular surgery when IOP needs to be decreased. Mannitol is available in 5% to 25% solution for injection. Dosage, concentration, and rate of administration must be individualized for its intended use and effect.

Prostaglandin Analogues

Certain prostaglandins have a role in elevating IOP, while others have the ability to lower it. Prostaglandin analogues mimic prostaglandins. Prostaglandin analogues (Table 11-1) increase the outflow of aqueous. The increased drainage occurs in the suprachoroidal space behind the iris, as opposed to the trabecular meshwork. This mode of outflow has proven extremely effective.

Latanaprost 0.005% (Xalatan®) was the first approved prostaglandin analogue. Research shows that it is more effective than the beta blockers at lowering pressure, and it has fewer side effects. One drop of latanaprost is used each night, which may increase compliance over the twice-daily beta blockers. The manufacturer recommends that this therapeutic be kept refrigerated until it is opened and kept at room temperature thereafter.

Prostaglandins have the ability to increase inflammation in the eye. Clinically relevant ocular inflammation has not been shown with use of latanaprost. However, surgeons generally avoid its use in postoperative patients due to a slightly increased risk of cystoid macular edema (CME). Second, prostaglandin analogues cause ocular redness, which is most pronounced 30 minutes after use and dissipates within an hour and a half. (Of course, if the drop is used at bedtime, this is inconsequential.) Finally, and most intriguing, approximately 3% of patients with light-colored irises have noticed increased iris pigmentation to the degree that eye color is changed. This event is benign but may be permanent. Latanaprost, with its greater efficacy, reduced side effects, and once-daily use, has overtaken beta blockers as the drug of choice for glaucoma therapy.

What the Patient Needs to Know

- Beta blockers can cause decreased heart rate, shortness of breath, and impotence. Inform your doctor if you think this is occurring.

- Miotics such as pilocarpine may cause headache, brow ache, and blurred vision when you first start using them. These symptoms usually decrease as you continue use.

- Miotics cause pupils to look very small.

- Carbonic anhydrase inhibiting drugs cause a metallic chalky taste and tingling in the fingers and toes.

- Hyperosmotics taste very sweet and should be sipped slowly.

- Latanaprost may cause the iris (colored part of the eye) to darken.

- Latanaprost should be refrigerated before opening but can be kept at room temperature thereafter.

Bibliography

Ajamian P, et al, eds. The do's and don'ts of taking glaucoma medication. *Foresight.* Otsuka American Pharmaceutical, Inc: 1996; 2(3).

Amoils SP. Phospholine iodine for control of hyperopia following RK. *Ocular Surgery News.* 1996;14(9):59.

Bartlett JD, Jaanus SD. *Clinical Ocular Pharmacology.* 2nd ed. Boston, Mass: Butterworths; 1989.

Bijlefeld M. Biotechnology: Glaucoma drug developments. *Eye Care Technology Magazine.* 1996;6(2):36-39.

Cantor LB. *Longterm safety and efficacy of brimonidine 0.2% and timolol 0.5% in glaucoma and ocular hypertension.* The Brimonidine Study Group. Abstract. Supplied by Allergan Pharmaceuticals.

Catania LJ. *Primary Care of the Anterior Segment.* East Norwalk, Conn: Appleton & Lange; 1990.

Dirks M. *Long-term safety and IOP-lowering efficacy of brimonidine tartrate 0/2% in glaucoma and ocular hypertension.* The Brimonidine Study Group. Abstract. Supplied by Allergan Pharmaceuticals.

Friedlander M, Bartlett J. Pullout guide to glaucoma drugs. *Eye Care Technology Magazine.* 1996;6(2):23-25.

Iwach A. Drug treatment for glaucoma. *Eye Care Technology Magazine.* 1994; 4(2):52-55,108.

Kronemyer B. Rethinking medical management of glaucoma. *Primary Care Optometry News.* 1996;1(6):6.

Lewis LL, Fingeret M. *Primary Care of the Glaucomas.* East Norwalk, Conn: Appleton and Lange; 1993.

Lewis TL, et al. *Care of Patient with Open Angle Glaucoma: Optometric Clinical Practice Guideline.* American Optometric Assoc: 1995.

Mandel M. Timolol hemihydrate as safe and effective as Timoptic. *Primary Care Optometry News.* 1996; 1(6):8.

Marielo EN. *Human Anatomy & Physiology*. Redwood City, Calif: Benjamin/Cummings Publishing; 1989.

Melton R, Thomas R. *4th Annual Guide to Therapeutic Drugs*. Norwalk, Conn: Optometric Management; May 1995.

Moses RA, Hart W Jr. *Adler's Physiology of the Eye: Clinical Application*. 8th ed. St. Louis, Mo: CV Mosby; 1987.

One on one: New drugs, new options for glaucoma therapy. *Primary Care Optometry News*. 1996; 1(6):1,17-18.

Onofrey BE. *Clinical Optometric Pharmacology and Therapeutics*. Philadelphia, Pa: JB Lippincott; 1992.

Ophthalmic Drug Facts. St. Louis, Mo: JB Lippincott; 1990.

PDR for Ophthalmology. 23rd ed. Montvale, NJ: Medical Economics; 1995.

Physicians' Desk Reference (49th Edition, 23rd Edition for ophthalmology, 16th Edition for nonprescription drugs). Oradell, NJ: ER Barnhardt/Medical Economics; published annually.

Rosenthal XL, Walters T, Berg E, Safyan E, Batoosingh AL. A comparison of safety and efficacy of brimonidine 0.2%, bid vs. tid, in subjects with elevated intraocular pressure. *Ophthalmology Clinical Research*. Austin, Tex and St. Louis, Mo: Allergan, Inc; 1996. Abstract. Supplied by Allergan Pharmaceuticals.

Silverman HM, ed. *The Pill Book*. 6th ed. New York, NY: Bantam Books; 1994.

Chapter 12

Side Effects, Toxicity, and Hypersensitivity

Ocular Side Effects of Systemically Administered Medications

It has been said that the eye is the bellwether of the body politic. Simply put, what goes on elsewhere in the body can exert effects that are visible in the eye. For the purposes of this discussion, we should acknowledge that it is almost impossible to take any medication without it having some side effect somewhere in the body. As the eye receives a continuous high-flow blood supply, it is commonly subject to toxicity from systemically administered medications.

There are several classes of drugs that are specifically known to have ocular toxicity. In clinical practice, the 2 medications that result in referral for ophthalmic evaluation are prednisone and chloroquine. Chemotherapy will also be discussed briefly.

Prednisone is administered for conditions such as asthma, arthritis, skin problems, and immunosuppression. Far and away, most medication-caused ocular side effects will be due to prednisone usage. The 2 most common ocular side effects of systemic or topical corticosteroids are increased IOP (glaucoma) and posterior subcapsular cataracts.

Chloroquine (Plaquenil®) is used in individuals with collagen vascular diseases such as arthritis and lupus. It has been known to accumulate in pigmented tissues within the body and can concentrate within the eye in such tissues as the cornea and the retinal pigment epithelium. Corneal deposition of chloroquine rarely has visual implications. However, deposition of the drug within the retina can lead to loss of night vision and progressive deterioration of central visual acuity.

Chemotherapeutic agents can cause conjunctivitis, ocular inflammation, and edema. In addition, systemic chemotherapy can induce a dry eye syndrome. All patients who are undergoing chemotherapy should use ocular lubricants and be observed closely by their eyecare professionals.

What the Patient Needs to Know

- Make sure every doctor who sees you has a complete list of all your medications, including OTC ones.

- Keep a list of your drug allergies.

- Any medication you take can have side effects.

- If you feel that you are having a reaction to a medication, call your physician.

- Signs of severe drug reaction are difficulty breathing, change in heart rate, light-headedness, rash, nausea, vomiting, and diarrhea. Seek medical attention at once.

Side Effects in Ocular Structures

Cornea

All antibiotics will have some side effect on the eye. The aminoglycosides, when used for extended periods of time, can lead to corneal epithelial breakdown and keratopathy. Swelling of the cornea has been seen with oral contraceptive use. Phenylbutazone can cause keratitis. Depositions of drugs in the cornea may occur with the use of chloroquine, amiodarone, chlorpropamide, clofazimine, gold salts, indomethacin, phenothiazines, and Vitamin D. When deposition of gold occurs (as in an individual who is taking systemic gold for arthritis), fine crystals, known as ocular chrysiasis, can be seen in the corneal epithelium and anterior stroma.

Conjunctiva

Conjunctival inflammation and follicular proliferation can occur when antibiotics are used. Other drugs that can induce conjunctivitis are barbiturates, chloral hydrate, guanethidine, methyldopa, methysergide, phenylbutazone, and sulfonamides. Gold salts, clofazemine, phenothiazine, quinacrine, Vitamin A, Vitamin D, and epinephrine can result in conjunctival deposits. A Stevens-Johnson type syndrome with inflammation of the mucous membranes can occur with barbiturates, chlorpropamide, and sulfonamide usage.

Extraocular Muscles

Disruption of muscular function causing nystagmus can be seen with gold salts, diazepam, ketamine, oral contraceptives, phenytoin, and salicylates. Frank paralysis of muscles can occur with penicillamine, phenytoin, chlorpropamide, anesthetics, and curarelike substances. Ptosis of the upper eyelid has also been associated with barbiturates, guanethidine, and penicillamine.

Anterior Segment

IOP can increase with topical, peribulbar, and systemic use of corticosteroids such as prednisone and prednisolone. In addition, increased IOP is associated with nonsteroidal anti-inflammatory drugs (NSAIDs), amphetamines, and anticholinergic agents, such as atropine and tricyclic antidepressants that have an atropinelike action.

Intraoperative floppy iris syndrome (IFIS) has been reported in men who are taking tamsulosin HCL (Flomax®) for benign prostatic hyperplasia. The systemic effect of this potent alpha$_{1A}$ antagonist is to relax the bladder neck. It also acts on the iris dilator muscle to cause atrophy and akinesia, resulting in a poorly dilating, floppy iris. It is important that the ophthalmic history includes asking about Flomax use in any male considering intraocular surgery.

Lens

The most common side effect of prednisone is posterior subcapsular cataracts. Increased risk of cataract development has been reported in the cholesterol-lowering agent Mevacor® although actual clinical cases are quite uncommon. Allopurinol, busalfan, and haloperidol have also been associated with cataract formation. The same drugs that cause pigmentation deposition in the cornea can also be deposited on the anterior surface of the lens, as is seen with gold salts and phenothiazine.

Optic Nerve

Optic atrophy can result from glaucoma induced by corticosteroids or by the direct action of barbiturates, chloramphenicol, iodoquinol, and MAO inhibitors. Inflammation of the nerve (neuritis) has been associated with chloramphenicol, disulfiram, ethambutol, isoniazid, morphine, penicillamine, rifampin, and streptomycin. Swelling of the optic nerve, as is seen in increased intracranial pressure (papilledema), can be associated with chlorambucil, nalidixic acid, oral contraceptives, tetracycline, and Vitamin A.

Retina

Macular degeneration syndromes can occur with the use of cardiac glycosides, chloroquine, and phenothiazinc. Retinal edema has been associated with oral contraceptives. Retinal hemorrhage has been seen as a result of anticoagulant, phenylbutazone, salicylate, or sulfonamide use. Changes in the vascular pattern have been reported with hexamethonium, oral contraceptives, and quinine.

Sildenafil citrate (Viagra®) and the family of erectile dysfunction drugs (Cialis®, Levitra®) taken orally are associated with blue/green color impairment (erythropsia). Although the effect is temporary, it may be disturbing, and patients on these drugs should be informed.

OphA OphT Systemic Effects of Topically Administered Ocular Medications

Any topically administered medication can enter the body system as a whole. First, topical eye medication can be absorbed into the body directly through the mucosal membranes of the eye. A much larger dose, however, can drain through the lacrimal system into the nasal mucosa and can be swallowed, delivering a systemic dose of ocular medication. To avoid this "oral" dose, patients should be instructed to instill eye drops by using the "pouch technique": grasping the outer third of the eyelid with the thumb and index finger and forming a pocket. The eye drop is placed into the pocket, the eyelid is gently closed, and the excess is wiped away. This technique prevents activation of the blink mechanism and lacrimal pump, which avoids sucking the medication through the lacrimal system into the nose. If the patient reports that he or she tastes the eye medicine, apply gentle pressure to the lacrimal sac with the finger after putting in the drop. Virtually all topically applied medications are capable of producing allergic reactions, including anaphylaxis.

Any medication that has an effect on the autonomic nervous system, such as direct-acting miotics, can cause flushing, bradycardia, and low blood pressure. Atropinelike drugs such as homatropine or scopolamine, which block the effects of acetylcholine, can cause confusion, dermatitis, dryness of the mouth, hyperexcitability, red skin, fever, psychotic episode and hallucinations, fast heart rate, and excessive thirst. All of these autonomic system side effects can be seen with as little as 1 drop instilled into the eye.

The most common topically administered ocular drugs causing systemic side effects are the epinephrinelike compounds used to dilate the pupil. These drugs can be rapidly absorbed through the mucosal membranes of the eye, leading to increased blood pressure and rapid heart rate. Periocular injection of anesthetics combined with epinephrine can cause the same effects quite rapidly, leading to respiratory collapse and even death.

The parasympathomimetic drugs, such as pilocarpine and carbachol, can cause cramping, diarrhea, low blood pressure, excessive salivation, nausea, lightheadedness, tremors, difficulty breathing, excessive sweating, and lethargy.

The most serious complications of topical antibiotic use include severe allergic reaction, which can occur with virtually any antibiotic. Aplastic anemia has been reported with chloramphenicol and can be life-threatening. Some individuals experience depigmentation of the eyelids, gastrointestinal side effects, and dermatitis. Chlortetracycline and tetracycline have been associated with skin discoloration, redness, and excessive light sensitivity. These 3 antibiotics are all topical.

Antiviral agents such as idoxuridine, trifluridine, and vidarabine have been associated with contact dermatitis, allergic reactions, and corneal epithelial breakdown with conjunctivitis. Neomycin can induce severe allergic reactions including dermatitis, redness of the skin, and itching. This reaction may occur systemically as well as in the periorbital region.

Although their use is less widespread today than in previous years, the sulfa drugs, such as sulfacetamide and sulfisoxazole, can lead to severe dermatitis in susceptible individuals who are allergic to sulfa. The drug can cause increased photosensitivity, Stevens-Johnson type syndrome of mucous membrane inflammation, and abnormalities in the blood profile. These blood abnormalities can be severe enough to require hospitalization.

Topical beta blockers can lead to cardiac arrhythmias, difficulty in breathing, slow heart rate, confusion, dizziness, upset stomach and gastrointestinal disturbances, headache, low blood pressure, and rashes.

Any time an individual develops side effects from any medication, the drug should be discontinued and the patient should be evaluated. It should be assumed that a side effect is the result of either ocular or systemic medication when the timing of the symptoms are closely associated with the commencement of medication use. Because there are potential cross reactions between different medications, patients should report any and all medications that they are taking, either ocular or systemic, to each physician who examines them. It is helpful to provide patients with a list of the ocular medications, their dosages, and potential side effects so that they can report these medications to their general physician. Once any allergic reaction has occurred, the patient should be provided with a card that lists the drug and the reaction.

A comprehensive listing of all potential interactions is beyond the scope of this book. We suggest the reader consult the *Physicians' Desk Reference of Drug Side Effects* for detailed information on various drugs. Suffice it to say here that before any patient is given medication, the practitioner must conduct a thorough investigation of the drug's potential side effects and possible interactions with other medications.

Chapter 13

Retinal Therapies

KEY POINTS

- There are 2 forms of age-related macular degeneration (AMD): the dry and wet types. Wet AMD usually requires treatment.

- Patients with retinal disease are at high risk of losing vision and should be monitored very closely.

- Patients who are treated for retinal bleeding can have serious drug-related side effects.

- Examiners should be alert to and consider any change in vision as significant.

The leading cause of blindness in the developed world is age-related macular degeneration (AMD). Affecting over 13 million people in the United States alone, it leads to significant morbidity (disability, expenses related to the illness, as well as the experience of the illness itself) and economic loss. As it affects individuals in the fifth to eighth decade of life, its effects on limiting vision as well as the threat of potential blindness can be devastating. There are 2 types of AMD: the relatively benign form known as dry AMD and the advanced form known as wet AMD. Wet AMD usually requires treatment.

Until recently, the ophthalmic community could do little more than diagnose AMD by identifying the hallmark drusen and pigmentary changes seen in the retina of affected individuals. The Age-Related Eye Disease Study (AREDS), sponsored by the National Eye Institute, determined that susceptible individuals could benefit early in the disease by taking a combination of antioxidant vitamins and changing their diets (see Appendix B). Fortunately, extensive work within the ophthalmic scientific community and partnerships with the pharmaceutical industry have recently led to the FDA approval of 2 new forms of treatment for these diseases (see below). These new treatments for AMD and other retinal vascular disorders offer hope for the millions of people who would otherwise have to accept the loss of their sight. In addition, there are presently several new drugs under development that will similarly improve the outlook for individuals with retinal disease.

Visudyne

Verteporfin (Visudyne®, manufactured by Novartis) is used with a special laser light to seal abnormal blood vessel formation and leakage in the retina that, untreated, can lead to loss of eyesight. It is indicated for the following conditions:

- Pathologic myopia with associated abnormal blood vessels or bleeding.
- Ocular histoplasmosis.
- Macular degeneration.

This medication is administered by intravenous injection. Treatment with verteporfin and laser light occurs in 2 steps. First, the verteporfin is injected. Then, 15 minutes later, a laser light is directed into the affected eye to activate the drug where it is needed. In some cases, more than 1 treatment session may be required. Verteporfin is less effective in patients 75 years of age or older.

When using verteporfin, it is especially important that the health care professional know about medications that could interfere with the drug (Table 13-1). A thorough health history is essential.

After receiving an injection of verteporfin, the eyes and skin will be extra sensitive to light, including sunlight and bright indoor lights. Certain types of sunglasses can help protect the eyes. *Do not expose the skin to direct sunlight or to bright indoor lights during this time*. Sunscreens will *not* protect the skin from a severe reaction to light (blistering, burning, and swelling). However, exposure to normal amounts of indoor light (eg, daylight or light from lamps with shades) will help clear the verteporfin from the skin. Therefore, *do not avoid normal amounts of indoor light*.

Commonly, patients being treated with Visudyne may experience headache and blurred vision, other changes in vision, bleeding, blistering, burning, coldness, discoloration of skin,

Table 13-1
Drug Interactions With Visudyne

Calcium channel blocking agents (medicine class for blood pressure)

Polymyxin B (antibiotic in eye preparations)

Radiation therapy (use of these medicines with verteporfin may increase the effects of verteporfin)

Alcohol

Antioxidant vitamins and minerals (eg, Beta-carotene)

Dimethyl sulfoxide (eg, DMSO, Rimso-50)

Medications that decrease blood clotting

Oral diabetes medication (may decrease the effects of verteporfin and blood vessel constriction)

Griseofulvin (eg, Fulvicin, Gris-PEG)

Phenothiazines (antipsychotic medications)

Sulfonamides

Tetracyclines

Rhiazide diuretics

Previous reaction to verteporfin (reaction is more likely to occur again)

feeling of pressure, infection, itching, numbness, pain, rash, redness, scarring, stinging, swelling, tenderness, tingling, ulceration, and/or warmth at the injection site. Less common side effects include decrease in vision (may be severe); dizziness; nervousness; eye pain; fainting; fast, slow, or irregular heartbeat; itching, redness, or other irritation of eye; pale skin; pounding in the ears; trouble breathing on exertion; unusual bleeding or bruising; unusual tiredness or weakness; back pain (during infusion of verteporfin); chills; cloudy urine; constipation; cough; decreased hearing; decreased sensitivity to touch; diarrhea; difficult or painful urination; and/or difficulty in moving.

Macugen

Recently, the FDA approved a novel approach to the treatment of abnormal blood vessels in the eye. Extensive study has demonstrated that a secreted protein known as Vascular Endothelial Growth Factor (VEGF) selectively binds and activates receptors located primarily on the surface of vascular endothelial cells. VEGF induces new abnormal vessel formation (angiogenesis) and increases vascular permeability and inflammation, all of which are thought to contribute to the progression of the neovascular (wet) form of AMD.

Pegaptanib sodium injection (Macugen®, manufactured jointly by Pfizer and Eyetech) is a selective VEGF antagonist. The first targeted anti-VEGF therapy, Macugen works differently from other currently available treatments for neovascular (wet) AMD. This drug is injected directly into the vitreous cavity of the eye and requires multiple repeat injections to be effective. Its action is to slow down or halt new vessel growth, which would otherwise increase the risk of intraocular bleeding. After intravitreous administration, Macugen mainly remains within the vitreous fluid, retina, and aqueous fluid and acts directly within the eye.

The major potential side effects of Macugen therapy relate to its method of administration. By injecting the drug directly into the eye, there is the risk of endophthalmitis. Proper aseptic injection technique should always be utilized when administering Macugen. Patients should be monitored during the week following injection for any signs of infection, pain, or loss of vision. There also have been reports of increased IOP within 30 minutes of injection. Therefore, IOP and the appearance of the optic nerve should be monitored and treated, if necessary.

Diabetic retinopathy is the leading cause of vision loss in individuals in affluent societies who are less than 50 years of age. Macugen is also being studied for its effectiveness in patients with diabetic macular edema as well as with retinal vein occlusion.

In addition to Macugen, Lucentis (ranibizumab, Genentech Inc), will probably gain FDA approval in the near future. The mode of administration and method of action as a VEGF inhibitor of these newer entries are similar. Preliminary clinical trials with slightly different dosing with Lucentis show promise.

Bibliography

Ambati J, Ambati BK, Yoo SH, Ianchulev S, Adamis AP. Age-related macular degeneration: etiology, pathogenesis, and therapeutic strategies. *Surv Ophthalmol.* 2003;48:257-293.

D'Amore PA. Mechanisms of retinal and choroidal neovascularization. *Invest Ophthalmol Vis Sci.* 1994;35:3974-3979.

Witmer AN, Vrensen GFJM, Van Noorden CJF, Schlingemann RO. Vascular endothelial growth factors and angiogenesis in eye disease. *Prog Retin Eye Res.* 2003;22:1-29.

Zarbin MA. Current concepts in the pathogenesis of age-related macular degeneration. *Arch Ophthalmol.* 2004;122:598-614.

Acute Drug Reactions and Emergencies

By nature, a medical practice has a diverse patient population with a wide array of physical and mental conditions. As a result, emergencies—ophthalmic and non-ophthalmic alike—can and will occur. Quick thinking and a trained response by both doctor and staff can prevent possible tragic consequences.

Emergency phone numbers for fire, police, poison control, and emergency medical services should be posted conspicuously at every phone. In many areas, these services can be universally obtained by dialing 911.

First, it is imperative that all medical office personnel become comfortably familiar with the emergency protocols established by the doctor. Everyone should know where first aid supplies and instruments are stored. Many offices have a special kit or crash cart readily available in case of emergency. These often contain a myriad of supplies and pharmaceuticals including epinephrine, cortisone, oxygen, and syringes. An emesis basin, smelling salts, and irrigating solutions should also be readily available.

Proper emergency response necessitates that all staff have a basic knowledge of first aid and CPR and be prepared to act, if necessary. Training in these areas is available through community organizations like the American Red Cross.

Acute drug reactions can arise following administration of any drug by any route. Such reactions are much more likely to occur following systemic administration and are rarely seen following topical administration. Acute drug reactions may be due to overstimulation of the central nervous system or a result of allergic reaction (anaphylaxis). Though normally not serious, acute drug reactions can be fatal and must always be considered emergencies.

Anaphylaxis is a potentially deadly hypersensitivity that can result from any drug. Patients with a medical history of hives, hay fever, and asthma are at greatest risk of developing anaphylaxis. Signs of such an acute allergic reaction are itching and rash, difficulty breathing, and a rapid, weak pulse. These problems usually start within 20 to 30 minutes of drug administration. It has been reported that patients who go on to develop life-threatening complications often report a deep generalized burning sensation or pain. If a patient complains of or begins exhibiting any of these signs or symptoms, it should be brought to the physician's attention without delay so that precautionary or therapeutic measures can be instituted. The treatment for anaphylaxis may include epinephrine, cortisone, and oxygen. Know how to respond and where to find the necessary medical supplies. Delays can be tragic.

In addition to acute drug reactions, emergency situations occur for a number of other reasons, including poor health, decreased peripheral awareness, and loss of strength and coordination. Fainting, falling, chest pain, difficulty breathing, and acute allergic reactions are likely to be encountered. Tightness or pain in the chest, breathing difficulties, and seizures should be considered serious and life-threatening and reported immediately for proper evaluation. Always be alert and watch the patient for clues that there is a problem. Pallor, unsteadiness, pain, faintness, nausea, extreme fatigue, or a "need to lie down" should signal the doctor and staff to watch that patient closely.

If a patient falls in the office, the doctor should be notified immediately. The victim should not be moved until the doctor completes a full assessment of the situation and patient's status. Fainting is a common cause of falls. A patient who feels faint should be placed with his or her head lower than the heart. If the patient does actually pass out, notify the doctor at once. Loosen the patient's collar or necktie. Smelling salts may be used to revive the patient. The patient should remain still until the dizzy feeling is gone. If the patient tries to stand up too soon, he or she may fall or pass out again. Be ready to assist. Once the patient has recovered, provide reassurance.

OptA

OphA

Srg

Vitamins

Sunlight, toxic environmental processes, and even normal metabolic activities can generate highly reactive molecules known as free radicals. These free radicals can damage surrounding cells and tissues. Antioxidant vitamins and minerals protect against injury caused by free radicals. There are over 200 antioxidants, including vitamins A, C, and E; beta-carotene; and minerals such as selenium and zinc.

Free radical formation has been implicated in a number of conditions, including cataracts, dry eye, and macular degeneration. The retina seems to be more susceptible to this damage than other tissues. Some studies suggest that the intake of antioxidant vitamins may help to delay the formation or slow the progress of these conditions. These relationships were extensively studied in a major multicenter clinical trial known as the Age-Related Eye Disease Study (AREDS). It was sponsored by the National Eye Institute, one of the federal government's National Institutes of Health. The AREDS set out to determine the natural history and risk factors of age-related macular degeneration (AMD) and cataract and to evaluate the effect of high doses of antioxidants and zinc on the progression of AMD and cataract.

Results from the AREDS showed that high levels of antioxidants and zinc significantly reduce the risk of advanced age-related macular degeneration (AMD) and its associated vision loss. These same nutrients had no significant effect on the development or progression of cataract.

Supplements

Who should take the AREDS formulation? Those individuals who are at high risk for developing advanced AMD with either intermediate AMD (the presence of either many medium-sized drusen or 1 or more large drusen in 1 or both eyes) or advanced AMD in 1 eye but not the other eye should take the formulation, a combination of antioxidants plus zinc. Advanced AMD is defined as either a breakdown of light-sensitive cells and supporting tissue in the central retinal area (advanced dry form) or the development of abnormal and fragile blood vessels under the retina (wet form) that can leak fluid or bleed. Either of these forms of advanced AMD can cause vision loss.

Given the research findings, many practitioners are now recommending that their patients use antioxidant supplements and make dietary changes. Patients at risk should reduce fat in the diet, reduce overall caloric intake (reducing the risk of diabetes, one of the known risks for retinal disease), and eat more leafy green vegetables. The AREDS formulation included 500 milligrams of vitamin C, 400 international units of vitamin E, 15 milligrams of beta-carotene, 80 milligrams of zinc as zinc oxide, and 2 milligrams of copper as cupric oxide. (Copper was added to the AREDS formulations containing zinc to prevent copper deficiency, which may be associated with high levels of zinc supplementation.) Many supplements are currently available, including almost 30 specific brands targeted at the ophthalmic market and available without a prescription (Table B-1).

Supplement Toxicity

Patients and practitioners alike must understand that the benefits of these agents have been demonstrated but are in no way a substitute for a balanced diet. In addition, excessive amounts of antioxidants can lead to adverse effects. For example, excessive vitamin E can lead to muscle

---

Table B-1
Nutritional Supplements for the Eyes

Bilberry 2020	Eye Vites	MacuCaps	Oxy-Vision
Bright Eyes	FortifEye	Nutrivision	SEE
CataRx	I-CAPS	Ocucaps	Sightamins
Eyebright	Isight and I-Care	Ocucare	VisionFactors
Eye Formula	Itone	OcuDyne	VitalEyez
EyePower	Lipotriad	Ocuguard	VIZION
Eye Support	Lutein	Ocuvite	ZincACE

Compiled by Roy H. Rengstorff, OD, PhD. Used with permission.

---

weakness, fatigue, decreased thyroid function, and blurred vision. Too much zinc can lead to anemia. Smokers should avoid the use of beta-carotene. However, antioxidant therapy offers hope to patients with conditions (such as macular degeneration) that have very few preventative or therapeutic measures.

What the Patient Needs to Know

- Studies suggest that vitamin therapy is useful in slowing the development of cataracts, macular degeneration, and dry eye.

- "Eye vitamins" are not a replacement for a balanced diet. However, the increased doses in the vitamins exceed those that can be obtained through diet alone.

- It is possible to "overdose" on certain vitamins. Ask your eyecare practitioner or pharmacist to help you with the right amounts.

Most patients and many practitioners do not recognize that many so-called "over-the-counter food supplements" or herbal remedies have potential ocular toxicity. Home remedies, such as placing milk into the conjunctival cul-de-sac to make the eye "white" or lime juice to "clear the eye," also carry the risk of severe ocular injury to the uninformed. Here are some of the unexpected and common ocular side effects of herbal treatments and nutritional supplements (based upon case reports submitted to the FDA, the World Health Organization [WHO] and the National Registry of Drug-Induced Ocular Side Effects) published in the *American Journal of Ophthalmology*:

- *Canthaxanthine* has been found to cause abnormalities in static threshold perimetry,electroretinography, and dark adaptation.

- *Chamomile* may cause severe conjunctivitis when used in or around the eye. (Some have used the herb to treat styes and runny, irritated eyes.) It is also used to treat fevers, bronchitis, insomnia, indigestion, migraine headaches, inflammation, burns, and colds.

- *Datura* causes mydriasis (dilated pupils). It is used to treat bronchitis, coughs, influenza, asthma, and eye inflammation.

- *Echinacea purpurea* can lead to eye irritation and conjunctivitis with topical use. It is used to treat the common cold, urinary tract infections, coughs, burns, flu, and fevers.

- *Ginkgo biloba* can cause spontaneous hyphema and retinal hemorrhages. It has been pre-scribed for dementia, equilibrium disorders, peripheral occlusive arterial disease, asthma, tinnitus, hypertonia, angina pectoris, and tonsillitis.

- *Licorice* can cause pseudoaldosteronism (may feature headache, muscle weakness, sodium and water retention, decreased calcium level, high blood pressure, heart failure, and cardiac arrest) and transient visual loss after ingestion. It may also exacerbate migraine headaches. This herb has been used to treat upper respiratory tract infections, constipation, appendici-tis, hepatitis C, gastric ulcers, and peptic ulcers.

- *Niacin* can be associated with discoloration of the eyelids, decreased vision, dry eyes, cys-toid macular edema, loss of eyebrows and eyelashes, proptosis, eyelid edema, and superfi-cial punctate keratitis. It has been used for cerebrovascular and cardiovascular disease, schizophrenia, arthritis, hypertension, diabetes, sexual dysfunction, and migraine headaches.

- *Alternative forms of Vitamin A (retinol)*, such as tretinoin, isotretinoin, etretinate and acitretin, have been shown to cause intracranial hypertension. They are used for severe recalcitrant nodular acne, severe recalcitrant psoriasis, acne vulgaris, and to induce leukemia remission.

Bibliography

Age-related eye disease study--results. National Eye Institute. Available at: http://www.nei.nih.gov/amd/index.asp. Accessed May 21, 2005.

Fraunfelder FW. Ocular side effects from herbal medicines and nutritional supplements. *Am J Ophthalmol.* 2004;138(4):639-647.

Rengstorff RH. Antioxidants and dry eyes. Presented at International Vision Expo; March 31, 1996; New York, NY.

Seddon JM, Hennekens CH. Vitamins, minerals, and macular degeneration: promising but unproven hypoth-esis. *Archives of Ophthalmology.* 1994;112:176-178.

The Drug Approval Process

How do drugs get through the regulatory process of the FDA? A complete description of this complicated, expensive, and time-consuming process is beyond the scope of this book; however, there are some general guidelines that can make sense of this sometimes bewildering and confusing process.

The FDA was established by the United States Congress to protect the health and welfare of the American public from the introduction of unproven or potentially dangerous drugs. The process of drug approval starts with an application to the FDA, usually from a drug developer or pharmaceutical manufacturing company. The overall process from application to drug approval generally takes 7 to 12 years and can cost the drug manufacturer hundreds of millions of dollars beyond the development costs of the drug. The company is obligated to obtain the clinical data necessary to prove efficacy, demonstrate safety, and discover any potential side effects or dangers. It begins with a clinical trial that has 4 phases (I-IV).

Clinical trials represent a pre-market testing ground for unapproved drugs. During these trials, a drug that is about to undergo investigation is administered to humans and is evaluated for its safety and effectiveness in treating, preventing, or diagnosing a specific disease or condition. The results of these trials will comprise the single most important factor in the approval or disapproval of a new drug, according to the FDA.

The FDA Center for Drug Evaluation and Research (CDER) is the branch of the FDA responsible for evaluating these studies. CDER is responsible for both prescription and OTC drugs and is the largest of the FDA's 5 centers, with a staff of about 1,800 people.

The goal of clinical trials is to maintain safety and effectiveness in data collection, the most important consideration being the safety of the patients involved in these trials. The clinical trials are strictly monitored for their design and conduct to ensure the safety of the individuals that participate and that they are not exposed to unnecessary risks. The process advances according to the following:

Investigational New Drug Application

A drug sponsor submits an investigational new drug application (IND) to the FDA. Drug companies, research institutions, and others in the drug development business must provide results of preclinical testing in laboratory animals and the studies in which they plan to conduct human testing. The FDA will then decide whether the company may move forward with testing the drug on humans.

Clinical Trials

After approval of the IND by the FDA, the study sponsors must approach the local institutional review board (IRB) at the institution in which the proposed studies will be conducted. This institution is usually a hospital, medical center, or academic environment. The IRB is a group of doctors, nurses, and nonmedical people (clergy, lawyers, administrators) who oversee clinical research within that institution.

The IRB approves the clinical trial protocols, which describe the type(s) of people who may participate in the clinical trial, the schedule of tests and procedures, the medications and dosages to be studied, the length of the study, and the study's objectives. The IRB makes sure the study is acceptable to the institution, that participants have given consent and are fully informed of their risks, and that researchers take appropriate steps to protect patients from harm.

Phase 1 studies are usually conducted on healthy volunteers. This part of the study's goal is to determine the drug's most frequent side effects and how the drug is metabolized and excreted. The number of subjects typically ranges from 20 to 80. Safety is the end determinant of this phase.

Phase 2 studies begin if Phase 1 studies do not reveal unacceptable toxicity. While the emphasis in Phase 1 is on safety, the emphasis in Phase 2 is effectiveness. This phase determines whether the drug works in people who have a certain disease or condition. For controlled trials, patients receiving the drug are compared with similar patients receiving a different treatment—usually a placebo or a different drug. Typically, the number of subjects in Phase 2 studies ranges from a few dozen to about 300. Safety continues to be evaluated, and short-term side effects are studied.

Phase 3 studies begin if evidence of effectiveness is shown in Phase 2. These studies gather more information about safety and effectiveness, studying different populations and different dosages and using the drug in combination with other drugs. The number of subjects usually ranges from several hundred to about 3,000 people. At this stage, a drug manufacturer can make a new drug application to gain approval for marketing the drug.

Phase 4 studies occur after a drug is approved. These studies look at novel uses of the drug (other indications) or other populations. The long-term effects and how participants respond to different dosages are determined. Many times, a manufacturer can then apply for labeling, for other possible indications for the medication, or report to the FDA any unforeseen side-effects that were not determined in the initial clinical trials.

New Drug Application

This is the formal step required by a drug sponsor to have the FDA approve a new drug for marketing in the United States. A new drug application (NDA) includes all animal and human data on the drug as well as information about how the drug works, how a patient is administered the medication, and how the company will be manufacturing the compounds in the drug.

Bibliography

Drug applications. Center for Drug Evaluation and Research. Available at: http://www.fda.gov/cder/about/smallbiz/clinical_investigator.htm. Accessed: May 21, 2005.

Index

Printed in the United States